AF598111

CURRENT ISSUES IN THE DIAGNOSTICS AND TREATMENT OF ACUTE APPENDICITIS

Edited by **Dmitry Victorovich Garbuzenko**

Current Issues in the Diagnostics and Treatment of Acute Appendicitis
http://dx.doi.org/10.5772/intechopen.70917
Edited by Dmitry Victorovich Garbuzenko

Contributors

Fernando Meléndez, Jaime Fandiño, Alfredo Alvarado, Sung Il Choi, Sang Hyun Kim, Volkan Sarper Erikci, Dmitry Victorovich Garbuzenko

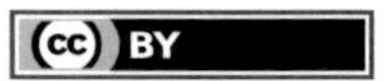

Notice

Statements and opinions expressed in the chapters are these of the individual contributors and not necessarily those of the editors or publisher. No responsibility is accepted for the accuracy of information contained in the published chapters. The publisher assumes no responsibility for any damage or injury to persons or property arising out of the use of any materials, instructions, methods or ideas contained in the book.

First published in London, United Kingdom, 2018 by IntechOpen
IntechOpen is the global imprint of INTECHOPEN LIMITED, registered in England and Wales, registration number: 11086078, The Shard, 25th floor, 32 London Bridge Street
London, SE19SG – United Kingdom
Printed in Croatia

British Library Cataloguing-in-Publication Data
A catalogue record for this book is available from the British Library

Additional hard copies can be obtained from orders@intechopen.com

Current Issues in the Diagnostics and Treatment of Acute Appendicitis, Edited by Dmitry Victorovich Garbuzenko
p. cm.
Print ISBN 978-1-78923-296-7
Online ISBN 978-1-78923-297-4

For EU product safety concerns:
IN TECH d.o.o., Prolaz Marije Krucifikse Kozulić 3, 51000 Rijeka, Croatia,
info@intechopen.com or visit our website at intechopen.com.

Meet the editor

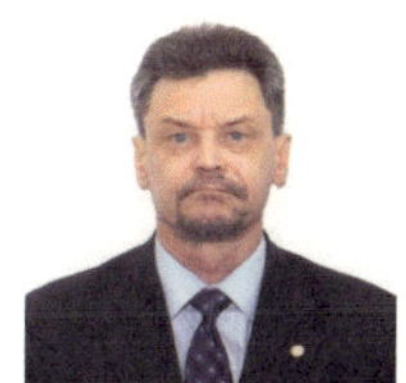

Dmitry Victorovich Garbuzenko graduated from Chelyabinsk State Medical Institute in 1985. From 1985 to 1987 he was a clinical intern. From 1987 to 1990 he was a postgraduate student of the Hospital Surgery Department in Chelyabinsk State Medical Academy. In 1991, he defended his PhD degree thesis. He was an assistant at the Department of Hospital Surgery from 1991 to 1996. In 1996 he became an assistant, then an associate professor (2003), and a professor (2006) at the Department of Surgery, South Ural State Medical University. In 2008 he defended his doctoral degree thesis (M.D.). Professor D.V. Garbuzenko is a member of the Russian Society of Surgeons. His practical activities associate with emergency abdominal surgery. He is the author of nearly 150 publications.

Contents

Preface

The book *Current Issues in the Diagnostics and Treatment of Acute Appendicitis* is devoted to the actual and in some cases controversial and unresolved problems associated with acute appendicitis, as well as peculiarities of its clinical picture, diagnosis, and treatment in children.

Acute appendicitis is one of the most common diseases in urgent surgery. About 100 years ago, S.I. Spasokukotsky, a famous Russian surgeon, said "So much has been spoken and written about acute appendicitis that it feels embarrassing when you try to encourage somebody to take notice of this issue." Despite these words, it is still the subject of attention among specialists around the world. Diagnosis of acute appendicitis, as in the old days, is based first of all on complaints, anamnestic data, and results of physical examination. Changes in laboratory parameters are unspecific but can be a good help in verification of the diagnosis, as well as imaging techniques. Nevertheless, their role continues to be discussed. In addition, various diagnostic scores have been proposed for this purpose, but none of them has been universally accepted. Surgical treatment of acute appendicitis in both adults and children has undergone a paradigm shift from open to laparoscopic appendectomy. In the last decade, antibiotic therapy is actively offered as an alternative in uncomplicated cases. In addition, the time of the operation and the safety of its delay in the hospital are discussed. Also, the subject of discussion is the management of patients in postoperative period. I believe that the materials of the book will be of interest to anyone who considers emergency abdominal surgery their specialty.

Professor Dmitry Victorovich Garbuzenko
Department of Faculty Surgery
South Ural State Medical University
Chelyabinsk, Russia

Section 1

Introduction

Chapter 1

Introductory Chapter: Controversies in the Diagnostics and Management of Acute Appendicitis

Dmitry Victorovich Garbuzenko

Additional information is available at the end of the chapter

http://dx.doi.org/10.5772/intechopen.76866

1. Introduction

Acute appendicitis is one of the most common diseases in urgent surgery. Despite this, it is not always easy to diagnose it, even for experienced surgeons. Acute appendicitis should be suspected in any patient with abdominal pain, and its correct diagnosis in many cases depends on the completeness of anamnestic data.

There are no other diseases that have such a variety of symptoms as acute appendicitis. At the same time, if gangrene develops, it may be asymptomatic until complications occur. And who among the surgeons have not ever observed the typical classic symptom complex and at the same time the absence of visual morphological changes in the appendix, after removal of which the patient felt better in the next few hours after the operation? In short, atypical acute appendicitis is more frequent than its classical manifestations.

2. Natural history and clinical assessment

As a rule, the main sign of acute appendicitis is abdominal pain, which makes a patient visit the doctor. It should be emphasized that the pain does not always occur in the right iliac fossa being the most typical position of the appendix. It may be in the epigastric region or migrate throughout the abdomen without any specific localization. In the initial period, pain is not intense, dull, and only occasionally may be cramping. After 2–3 h from the onset of the disease, they gradually increase and move to the right iliac region where the appendix is localized. This pain displacement is characteristic of acute appendicitis onset and is known as Kocher-Volkovich sign. This sign results from the initial pain signals being transferred

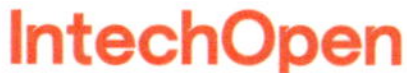

through the midgut visceral innervation. When the parietal peritoneum starts being involved in the inflammatory process, the pain acquires more certain localization.

Often patients mistakenly associate the presence of abdominal pain with an unhealthy diet or believe that they have got poisoned, especially since the disease is accompanied by loss of appetite, nausea, and one- or two-time reflexive vomiting from the very beginning. Sometimes patients try to induce vomiting artificially or pump the stomach. Murphy, in 1904, first described vomiting and migration of colicky central abdominal pain to the right iliac fossa.

Cope described constipation in patients and their expectations of pain relief after defecation, which does not happen. Urination problems are rare.

A simple visual examination in the first few hours shows the doctor that the patient's condition is not worsened much. He is comparatively calm, moves actively, and sometimes holds on to his right side. Pulse rate typically increases and does not correspond to body temperature, which often remains normal and rises as destructive changes develop in the appendix.

Further examination is supposed to reveal three signs that characterize acute appendicitis: tenderness, muscular contraction, and skin hyperesthesia (Dieulafoy triad). Abdominal tenderness is the most typical sign of acute appendicitis. Visually, the movements of the right iliac region moderately lag during breathing. An attempt to take a deep breath, draw in a stomach, or make a cough causes an intensification of pain.

Palpation of the abdomen should be started from the left side, away from the pain area. Caressing counter-clockwise movements should gradually approach the right iliac region, where the patient may suddenly feel a sharp and intolerable pain. In some cases, its epicenter is McBurney's point, which was described by the author as follows: "…exactly between an inch and half and two inches from the anterior spinous process of the ileum on a straight line drawn from that process to the umbilicus" [1]. This point was assumed to match with the location of the inflamed appendix irritating the abdominal peritoneum over the T11 and T12 dermatome segment. Opposed to McBurney's original description, most textbooks mistakenly define the point as being one-third of the line from the anterior superior iliac spine to the umbilicus. Meanwhile, Lanz believed that "the McBurney's point has nothing to do with the origin of the vermiform appendix" and suggested its own localization that is on the line between the two anterosuperior iliac spines one-third of the distance from the right spine [2].

In general, the projection of pain need not necessarily correspond to the Lanz or McBurney's point. Occasionally, pain is noted on the middle line under the umbilicus or above the pubic region. Less often it is found anteriorly or posteriorly in the right- or left hypochondrium. In the absence of pain in the surveyed areas, it is advised to turn a patient on the left side and palpate over the iliac crest and along its entire length. If a negative result is obtained, rectal examination should be started. Pain in the Douglas pouch is an excellent sign. It often combines with pain in the right iliac region but is often found singly.

Abdominal wall muscle contraction or defense (muscular protection) is the most important of the signs revealed on careful examination. According to Mondor, there is no other sign which allowed doctors to save more lives than this one. When palpating an abdomen, which is not swollen and rigid but does not participate in respiratory movements, it is necessary to attempt to find the reaction of the abdominal wall in the form of muscular contraction. In acute appendicitis, it is usually localized in the right iliac region. Skin hypersthesia appears in most cases of local or diffuse peritonitis [3].

In addition, there are many symptoms and signs that can be associated with appendicitis, depending on the location of the inflamed vermiform appendix, for example: Dunphy's sign (coughing intensifies pain in right lower quadrant), obturator sign (hip flexion and internal rotation increases pain), psoas sign (right hip passive extension increases pain in a patient lying on the left side), Rovsing's sign (palpation in the left lower quadrant intensifies pain in the right lower quadrant), etc. At the same time, most of them are not specific and their importance increases significantly when they are evaluated together with laboratory signs [4].

3. Laboratory values

Changes in laboratory parameters in acute appendicitis include leukocytosis with left shift and increased inflammatory markers such as C-reactive protein and erythrocyte sedimentation rate. As with the clinical symptoms and signs, each particular laboratory value hardly indicates the presence of acute appendicitis. However, combinations of clinical and laboratory data or aggregate of various laboratory values are more reliable. For example, it was determined that high rates of laboratory inflammatory markers such as white blood cell and granulocyte counts and C-reactive protein level were comparatively strong predictors of perforated appendicitis, whereas low values testified to its absence [5].

4. Scoring systems

There are several clinical scoring systems that are used to diagnose acute appendicitis. In 1986, Alfredo Alvarado developed his score, also called MANTRELS based on the mnemonic for remembering the combination of eight signs and symptoms: migration (1), anorexia-acetone (1), nausea-vomiting (1), tenderness in right lower quadrant (2), rebound pain (1), elevation of temperature (1), leukocytosis (2), shift to the left (1). Each indicator is assigned 1–2 points, which are then summed. If the sum of points equals numbers from 0 to 4, acute appendicitis is unlikely. The score of 5 or 6 means that acute appendicitis should be suspected and observation is necessary. The score of 7 and 8 signifies that the diagnosis is probable. Acute appendicitis is very likely if the score is 9 or 10 [6]. Currently, there have been developed the modified versions of the Alvarado scale, such as the Pediatric Appendicitis Score, described in 2002 by Samuel [7] and other scores such as the Eskelinen, Ohhmann, RIPASA scores [8], etc. Generally, these clinical scoring systems are more informative than specific symptoms or signs alone. Still, they are not capable of predicting appendicitis with sufficient probability and therefore should not be used alone to diagnose it. They have been applied to define the necessity for radiological tests or as a guide for planning clinical management.

5. Radiologic imaging

Radiological imaging is used more and more to evaluate abdominal pain and diagnose acute appendicitis. On one hand, imaging may be useful in the examination of patients with abdominal pain for establishing or excluding other diagnoses or for averting unnecessary surgery. On the other hand, imaging could possibly delay operation, and in the case of computed tomography (CT), radiologic imaging exposes patients to the risks of ionizing radiation. Abdominal ultrasound (US) is less and less used to diagnose acute appendicitis. It was designated that US sensitivity and specificity in this disease do not exceed those of physical examination or approved clinical scores such as the Alvarado score [9]. The noninvasive gold standard for acute appendicitis remains CT with contrast medium. It was proved that preoperative CT reduced the number of negative appendectomies but increased waiting time for surgery, although perforation rate was not elevated [10]. Magnetic resonance imaging (MRI) is a promising technique because of its high diagnostic accuracy and avoidance of ionizing radiation and intravenous contrast medium [11].

6. Management

Appendectomy is one of the most common surgical procedures performed worldwide. Since the late 1880s, open appendectomy has been accepted as the standard for the treatment of acute appendicitis and has saved many lives since then. In Europe, it was promoted by the thesis of Charles Krafft "Essay on the need for surgical treatment of perityphlitis and purulent perforated appendicitis" (1888), while in America there were the works of Charles McBurney, in particular, "Experience with early operative interference in cases of disease of the vermiform appendix" (1889) [12].

Treatment of uncomplicated acute appendicitis without surgery is principally unstudied, although it often resolves spontaneously or with antibiotic therapy. Few studies state that it has the outcomes comparable to those of appendectomy [13].

The widespread use of CT for the diagnosis of appendicitis led to interesting observations regarding the possibility of spontaneously resolved acute appendicitis. It was shown that the inclusion of the CT result in the Alvarado score increases the frequency of appendectomy. When classified as having a low likelihood of appendicitis (Alvarado score ≤ 4), patients who underwent a CT scan had an appendectomy rate of 48%. In contrast, those with an Alvarado score ≤ 4 who did not undergo a CT scan had an appendectomy rate of only 12% [14].

In another study, diagnostic laparoscopy was used instead of CT scan in the management of patients with nonspecific abdominal pain. Patients were randomized to either (1) diagnostic laparoscopy or (2) nonoperative management (with operative intervention if peritonitis developed). The appendectomy rate was 39% for those randomized to diagnostic laparoscopy and 13% for those managed nonoperatively [15].

In a number of studies, the incidence of acute uncomplicated appendicitis correlated strongly to the incidence of normal appendix removal and inversely correlated to diagnostic accuracy. Due to this, the authors reasoned that the observed incidence of uncomplicated appendicitis was influenced by the willingness to perform appendectomy in cases of presumed appendicitis. A high rate of appendectomy in such situations increases the proportion of confirmed cases probably by adding instances of self-limited inflammation that would escape detection in other circumstances [16]. This indirect evidence indicates that uncomplicated acute appendicitis can initially be treated without resorting to surgery. The safety of the initial non-surgical treatment of uncomplicated appendicitis was further confirmed, and it was shown that successful appendectomy can be avoided in almost all patients for the first 24 h with antibiotic therapy [17].

A large, population-based study using the American College of Surgeons National Surgical Quality Improvement Program database supports this semi-elective strategy, suggesting that appendectomy may be delayed up to 24–48 h without a significant increase in adverse outcome. In that study, there was no difference in the complication rate for those undergoing appendectomy within 1 day of admission. However, complication rate doubled if waiting time for surgery was delayed more than 48 h [18]. Contrary to the studies supporting a safe delay of appendectomy, there have been investigations demonstrating negative outcomes of even 6–12 h delays in surgery [19]. A recent study from the UK found no increased rate of complicated appendicitis when appendectomy was performed within 48 h [20].

7. Acute appendicitis in children

Acute appendicitis is one of the most common surgical diseases in children. It occurs in all age groups, but rarely in infants. The associated lethality is 0.1–1% with prevalence in young children. Death in infants and neonates happens because of: (1) the failure to identify the disease because of its clinical presentation, which is similar to other common conditions in this age group, and (2) the inability of a younger patient to tell about abdominal pain or the absence of systemic symptoms, such as fever. At the time of the diagnosis, the percentage of perforated appendicitis has been up to 30% [21]. The percentage of perforation has been stated as high as 80–100% for children younger than 3 years, compared with 10–20% in 10–17-year-old children [22].

In general, the strategy of diagnosis and treatment of acute appendicitis in children does not differ much from adults. Problems in the treatment of acute appendicitis are mostly the same in adults and children. Important concerns about the diagnosis, surgical technique, and antibiotic therapy remain uncertain for all patients. There are specific considerations for a pediatric appendectomy that remain questionable. They include the growing use of single-incision or single-port laparoscopic appendectomy and the primary nonoperative management of acute appendicitis with or without following appendectomy [23].

8. Conclusions

Acute appendicitis, being one of the most common diseases in emergency abdominal surgery, is a problem that still creates diagnostic difficulties. Although clinical studies alone cannot be sufficient to diagnose appendicitis, the importance of careful anamnesis and physical examination should not be underestimated. If extra tests are necessary, their risks and opportunities should be considered along with the possibility that such tests will change the management. Progress in imaging and computer decision support hold promise for the future, but additional study is needed to guarantee the accuracy, efficiency, and cost-effectiveness of novel diagnostic approaches for acute appendicitis.

The available data concerning nonoperative management of acute appendicitis is discrepant. Pathologic confirmation of appendicitis is one of the difficulties in performing a well-planned randomized clinical trial of nonoperative versus operative therapy for acute appendicitis. Successful antibiotic therapy for "suspected" appendicitis may cause doubts about the diagnosis. On the other hand, there are patients who undergo a negative appendectomy and surgical risks, which is a valid concern.

In spite of the fact that acute appendicitis is widespread, optimal diagnostics and management of it remain uncertain. This problem may be solved by conducting large multicenter randomized trials.

Author details

Dmitry Victorovich Garbuzenko

Address all correspondence to: garb@inbox.ru

Department of Faculty Surgery, South Ural State Medical University, Chelyabinsk, Russia

References

[1] McBurney C. Experience with early operative interference in cases of disease of the vermiform appendix. Northern New York Medical Journal. 1889;**50**:676-684

[2] Lanz O. Der McBurney'sche Punkt. Zentralblatt für Chirurgie. 1908;**35**:185-190

[3] Mondor H. Diagnostics Urgents, Abdomen. Paris, France: Edité par Masson & Cie; 1949

[4] Garbuzenko DV. Selected Lectures in Emergency Abdominal Surgery. Saarbrücken, Germany: LAP LAMBERT Academic Publishing GmbH& Co.; 2012

[5] Andersson RE. Meta-analysis of the clinical and laboratory diagnosis of appendicitis. The British Journal of Surgery. 2004;**91**(1):28-37

[6] Alvarado A. A practical score for the early diagnosis of acute appendicitis. Annals of Emergency Medicine. 1986;**15**(5):557-564

[7] Samuel M. Pediatric appendicitis score. Journal of Pediatric Surgery. 2002;**37**(6):877-881

[8] Erdem H, Çetinkünar S, Daş K, Reyhan E, Değer C, Aziret M, et al. Alvarado, Eskelinen, Ohhmann and Raja Isteri Pengiran Anak Saleha appendicitis scores for diagnosis of acute appendicitis. World Journal of Gastroenterology. 2013;**19**(47):9057-9062

[9] Giljaca V, Nadarevic T, Poropat G, Nadarevic VS, Stimac D. Diagnostic accuracy of abdominal ultrasound for diagnosis of acute appendicitis: Systematic review and meta-analysis. World Journal of Surgery. 2017;**41**(3):693-700

[10] Lietzén E, Salminen P, Rinta-Kiikka I, Paajanen H, Rautio T, Nordström P, et al. The accuracy of the computed tomography diagnosis of acute appendicitis: Does the experience of the radiologist matter? Scandinavian Journal of Surgery. 2018;**107**(1):43-47

[11] Cobben L, Groot I, Kingma L, Coerkamp E, Puylaert J, Blickman J. A simple MRI protocol in patients with clinically suspected appendicitis: Results in 138 patients and effect on outcome of appendectomy. European Radiology. 2009;**19**(5):1175-1183

[12] Williams GR. Presidential address: A history of appendicitis. With anecdotes illustrating its importance. Annals of Surgery. 1983;**197**(5):495-506

[13] Malik AA, Bari SU. Conservative management of acute appendicitis. Journal of Gastrointestinal Surgery. 2009;**13**(5):966-970

[14] Petrosyan M, Estrada J, Chan S, Somers S, Yacoub WN, Kelso RL, et al. CT scan in patients with suspected appendicitis: Clinical implications for the acute care surgeon. European Surgical Research. 2008;**40**(2):211-219

[15] Decadt B, Sussman L, Lewis MP, Secker A, Cohen L, Rogers C, et al. Randomized clinical trial of early laparoscopy in the management of acute non-specific abdominal pain. The British Journal of Surgery. 1999;**86**(11):1383-1386

[16] Howie JG, Cumming RL. The role of infection in transfusion thrombophlebitis. Lancet. 1962;**2**(7261):851-853

[17] Gandy RC, Wang F. Should the non-operative management of appendicitis be the new standard of care? ANZ Journal of Surgery. 2016;**86**(4):228-231

[18] Fair BA, Kubasiak JC, Janssen I, Myers JA, Millikan KW, Deziel DJ, et al. The impact of operative timing on outcomes of appendicitis: A National Surgical Quality Improvement Project analysis. American Journal of Surgery. 2015;**209**(3):498-502

[19] Teixeira PG, Sivrikoz E, Inaba K, Talving P, Lam L, Demetriades D. Appendectomy timing: Waiting until the next morning increases the risk of surgical site infections. Annals of Surgery. 2012;**256**(3):538-543

[20] United Kingdom National Surgical Research Collaborative, Bhangu A. Safety of short, in-hospital delays before surgery for acute appendicitis: Multicentre cohort study, systematic review, and meta-analysis. Annals of Surgery. 2014;**259**(5):894-903

[21] Ponsky TA, Huang ZJ, Kittle K, Eichelberger MR, Gilbert JC, Brody F, et al. Hospital- and patient-level characteristics and the risk of appendiceal rupture and negative appendectomy in children. Journal of the American Medical Association. 2004;**292**(16):1977-1982

[22] Pledger HG, Fahy LT, van Mourik GA, Bush GH. Deaths in children with a diagnosis of acute appendicitis in England and Wales 1980-4. British Medical Journal (Clinical Research Edition). 1987;**295**(6608):1233-1235

[23] Wray CJ, Kao LS, Millas SG, Tsao K, Ko TC. Acute appendicitis: Controversies in diagnosis and management. Current Problems in Surgery. 2013;**50**(2):54-86

Section 2

Acute Appendicitis: Diagnostic Problems and Debatable Questions of Management

Chapter 2

Clinical Approach in the Diagnosis of Acute Appendicitis

Alfredo Alvarado

Additional information is available at the end of the chapter

http://dx.doi.org/10.5772/intechopen.75530

Abstract

Abdominal pain is the most common reason for consultation in the emergency department, and most of the times, its cause is an episode of acute appendicitis. However, the misdiagnosis rate of acute appendicitis is high due to the unusual presentation of the symptoms. Therefore, the clinician has to be very alert in order to establish a correct diagnosis.

Keywords: diagnosis of acute appendicitis, clinical approach, Alvarado score

1. Introduction

The lifetime risk of appendicitis is 8.6% for males and 6.7% for females with an overall prevalence of 7% worldwide. The incidence of acute appendicitis has been declining steadily since the late 1940s, and the current annual incidence is 10 cases per 100,000 population. In Asian and African countries, the incidence of acute appendicitis is probable lower because of the dietary habits of the inhabitants of these geographic areas. Dietary fiber is thought to decrease the viscosity of feces, decrease bowel transit time, and discourage formation of fecaliths, which predispose individuals to obstructions of the appendicular lumen [1].

2. Epidemiology

There is a slight male preponderance of 3:2 in teenagers and young adults. In adults, the incidence of appendicitis is approximately 1.4 times greater in men than in women. However,

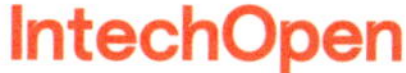

many studies have demonstrated a preponderance of female over male patients. The incident of primary appendectomy is approximately equal in both sexes [1].

The incidence of appendicitis gradually rises from birth, peaks in the late teen years, and gradually declines in the geriatric years. The mean age when appendicitis occurs in the pediatric population is 6–10 years. Lymphoid hyperplasia is observed more often among infants and young adults and is responsible for the increased incidence of appendicitis in those age groups. Younger children have a higher rate of perforation, with reported rates of 50–85%. The median age of appendectomy is 22 years. Although rare, neonatal and even prenatal appendicitis have been reported. Therefore, clinicians must maintain a high index of suspicion in all age groups [1]. According to Buckius et al. [2], in the USA the annual rate (per 10,000 population) of all cases of appendicitis and appendectomy increased from 7.62 in 1993 to 9.38 in 2008 and since then remained stable at 9.4 cases per 10,000. However, the ratio of simple appendectomy to complex cases has increased at extreme ages (0–9 and over 40 years). But in general, there is a trend in the percentage of complex cases that are decreasing from 33.4% in 1993 to 27% in 2008.

3. Etiology

The etiology of acute appendicitis is not quite clear. The main theory is that obstruction of the lumen of the appendix is the cause of acute appendicitis [3]. Fecalith, normal stool, and lymphoid hyperplasia are the main causes for obstruction. Obstruction probably plays a key role in the progression of appendicitis, but evidence for fecaliths as the most common cause of uncomplicated appendicitis is weak. Overall, fecaliths were found in 18.1% of appendicitis specimens and 28.6% of negative appendectomies. Fecaliths were associated with perforation more often than with uncomplicated appendicitis, and fecaliths are more common in pediatric cases than in adult appendicitis, independent of perforation [4].

4. Pathophysiology

The lumen distal to the obstruction starts to fill with mucus and acts as closed loop obstruction. This leads to distension and an increase in the intraluminal and intramural pressure. As the condition progresses, the resident bacteria in the appendix rapidly multiply [3]. Distension of the lumen of the appendix causes reflex anorexia, nausea and vomiting, and visceral pain. As the pressure of the lumen exceeds the venous pressure, the small venules and capillaries become thrombosed, but arterioles remain open, which lead to engorgement and congestion of the appendix. The inflammatory process soon involves the serosa of the appendix, hence the parietal peritoneum in the region, which causes classical right lower quadrant (RLQ) pain. Once the small arterioles are thrombosed, the area at the antimesenteric border becomes ischemic, and infarction and perforation ensue. Bacteria leak out through the dying walls, and pus forms within and around the appendix. Perforations are usually seen just beyond the obstruction rather than at the tip of the appendix [3].

http://dx.doi.org/10.5772/intechopen.75530

5. Diagnosis

The diagnosis of acute appendicitis is based on the history, physical examination, and laboratory investigation, as in any other disease [5]. Graff et al. [6] found that patients whose diagnosis was initially missed by the physician had fewer signs and symptoms of appendicitis that in patients who had more signs and symptoms initially. Older patients (>40 years old) had more false-negative decisions and a higher risk of perforation or abscess. On the other hand, false-positive decisions were made for patients who had signs and symptoms similar to those of appendicitis patients. They also found no increase in the perforation or abscess rate if the hospital delay was less than 20 hours. The normal appendix rate decreased from 15% to 1.9% after implementing an observation program, with no increase in perforation rate (26.7% before and 27.5% after).

The overall accuracy for diagnosing acute appendicitis is approximately 80% with a false-negative appendectomy rate of 20%. Diagnostic accuracy varies by sex, with a range of 78–92% in males and 58–85% in female patients. The morbidity from appendectomy showed steady improvement until 1962. Since that date, there has been a statistically significantly rise of morbidity reaching rates as high as 29%, but in the developing world, the rate is significantly higher [7]. Kong et al. reported a 60% perforation with a median duration from onset of symptoms of 4 days and an overall mortality of 1% [8]. Younger children have a higher rate of perforation with reported rates of 50–80%.

6. Medical history

The immediate history prior to the onset of pain is very important because frequently there is a history of indigestion, gastritis, or flatulence for a few days prior to the onset of pain. A history of unusual irregularity of the bowels is often obtained. Sometimes there is constipation, at other times diarrhea, especially in children [9].

Normally, appendicitis presents with highly characteristic sequence of symptoms and signs. Initially, appendicitis causes visceral pain poorly localized to the epigastrium or periumbilical region, presumably because of distension of the appendix. Anorexia, nausea, and vomiting soon follow as the pathology worsens. More advanced inflammation causes irritation of adjacent structures or the peritoneum, low-grade fever, and peritoneal pain localized in the right lower quadrant (RLQ). Pain usually occurs before vomiting, and the patient has usually not experienced similar symptoms before the present episode [10].

7. Family history

A careful family history should be obtained for every child in whom acute appendicitis is suspected [11]. A positive family history of acute appendicitis increases the risk by 3.18 times in a patient with acute abdominal pain, and the chance of appendicitis is 10 times greater in a child with at least one relative with reported appendicitis [12]. Retrocecal appendicitis has been reported in members of the same family in various countries [13]. Shperber et al. reported four members of the same family operated on for acute retrocecal appendicitis. In all four cases, there was pain or tenderness in the right lower quadrant of the abdomen accompanied by fever and leukocytosis. All of these cases support the hypothesis that a hereditary factor may be involved in the pathogenesis of acute appendicitis.

Therefore, a family history of acute appendicitis is an important factor to be taken into consideration during the medical interview [14]. Ethnic and geographical variations have been reported regarding the position of the appendix, and this variable anatomy may pose a challenge during appendectomy because it may necessitate extension of a transverse incision or additional muscle splitting [15].

8. Physical examination

The patient usually has a low-grade fever (<38°C) with associated tachycardia and appears flushed and with a dry tongue and fetor oris. The patient often lies still as movement and coughing exacerbate the pain. In children the hop test has been advocated as a test to confirm appendicitis. The child is asked to hop but refuses as this causes pain [15].

Before examining the abdomen, it is well to learn from the patient the exact place where the pain started, and if have been an alteration in its location. The exact location of maximal pain should be pointed out at the time of examination. Inspection of the abdomen will reveal at a glance any abnormal local or general distension and will in some cases determine the presence of a tumor or abdominal swelling. All the hernia orifices must be inspected as a routine and special attention directed to the femoral canal, where, in a fat subject, a small hernia is easy to overlook [9].

9. Symptoms and clinical signs

In an international systematical review of appendicitis scores, Ying-lie [16] found that the most common features are elevated whit blood count (WBC), right lower quadrant pain tenderness, combination of anorexia, nausea or vomiting, rebound tenderness, and migration of pain to the right lower quadrant. In 21 studies after 2000, polymorphonuclear leukocyte count (PMNC) was also relevant, and five studies included C-reactive protein (CRP).

Abdominal pain is the primary presenting complaint of patients with acute appendicitis. The diagnostic sequence of colicky central abdominal pain followed by vomiting with migration to the right iliac fossa is present in only 50% of patients. Loss of appetite is often a predominant feature. Constipation and nausea with profuse vomiting may indicate development of generalized peritonitis after perforation but is rarely a major feature in simple appendicitis. Male patients with a retrocecal appendix may complain of right testicular pain, and in some cases, in children, inflammation of the right scrotal area is present [17].

Migration of pain from the epigastric region or periumbilical area to the right lower quadrant, also known as the Volkovich-Kocher sign, is an important symptom at the beginning of the disease.

Right lower quadrant tenderness is the most common clinical sign which occurs in a great majority of patients with acute appendicitis. It has an 85% sensitivity and a 90% specificity with a positive likelihood ratio of 7.3:8.0 and a negative likelihood of 0:0.26.

Rebound pain (Blumberg sign) is one of the most useful signs of acute appendicitis in children even if it is sometimes difficult to elicit it, but with some practice and patience, it is possible to obtain a positive result. It is for this reason that some clinicians have proposed similar signs to replace rebound pain. For instance, Samuel [18] in his PAS score replaced cough, percussion tenderness, and hopping tenderness for rebound pain. Elevation of temperature (37.3°C), not fever, is present in the early stages of acute appendicitis, and in the late stages, it will progress into fever with temperatures above 37.7°C. Usually the increase of the temperature will run parallel to leukocytosis.

10. Other indirect signs of rebound pain

Rovsing sign is related to the rebound tenderness test and has to do with peritoneal irritation. The cough test, described by Rostovzev, known also as the Dunphy's sign, has a near-perfect sensitivity with a specificity of 95% for the detection of acute appendicitis. The Markle test (heel drop jarring) [19], pain on walking, pain with jolts, or bumps in the road are also signs of peritoneal irritation.

11. Uncommon tests in acute appendicitis

Psoas sign or Obraztsova's sign or the Cope's psoas test has a very low sensitivity (16%) but a good specificity (96%) and is present in retrocecal and pelvic appendix. It is elicited with the patient in the supine position, asking the patient to lift the right thigh against the examiner's hand placed just above the knee. Alternatively, with the patient in the left lateral decubitus position, the examiner extends the patient's right leg at the hip. Increased pain with either maneuver constitutes a positive sign [15].

According to Cope [9], the irritation and reflex rigidity of the iliopsoas muscle frequently cause the patient to hold the right thigh flexed, or with a lesser degree of irritation, the pain may be felt if the right thigh be fully extended as the patient lies on the left side. This sign is often of great value. The perforated pelvic appendix is one of the most easily overlooked and therefore one of the most dangerous conditions, which may occur in the abdomen. It is at least essential to diagnose the ruptured appendicitis as soon as possible after rupture before peritonitis has extended too far upward into the abdominal cavity. Irritation of the bladder or rectum may be signified by frequency or pain during micturition or by diarrhea or tenesmus, respectively.

Obturator sign is similar to the psoas sign. It is elicited by passively flexing the right hip and knee and internally rotating the leg at the hip, stretching the obturator muscle. Resultant right-sided abdominal pain is a positive sign, indicating irritation of the obturator muscle [15]. When the ruptured appendix is adherent to the fascia covering the obturator internus muscle, rotation of the flexed thigh will cause hypogastric pain. In performing this maneuver, it is essential that the thigh be flexed so as to relax the psoas muscle [9].

Uncommon signs are related to cutaneous hyperesthesia such as the discomfort in the "Sherren's" triangle (umbilicus-pubic tubercle-anterior superior iliac crest) in cases of early acute appendicitis. The Massouh sign [20] is a clinical sign for acute localized appendicitis that consists of swishing two finger tips starting on the xiphoid sternum down toward the left and right iliac fossae to elicit hyperesthesia due to peritoneal irritation. A positive sign is a grimace of the patient upon a right-sided (and not left) sweep. Also, lightly touching the patient with the stethoscope creates uncomfortable sensation on the affected area. These two tests can replace the migration symptom in children who cannot communicate well.

The K-sign has been named after its region of origin, Kashmir, and is present in retrocecal and paracolic appendicitis. It is elicited by percussion and palpation of the posterior abdominal wall and is present in patients of Indian ethnicity and coexists with the psoas sign. This sign is similar to the percussion test described in the MANTRELS score included in this chapter. The K-sign can lead to an early diagnosis of acute appendicitis localized in the retrocecal and retrocolic spaces [21].

The Hamburger sign is used for the diagnosis of appendicitis. The sign is used to rule out that disease, with the physician inquiring if the patient would like to consume his favorite food. If the patient wants to eat, the clinician should consider other diagnoses than appendicitis. This sign could replace the symptom of anorexia that is 80% sensitive for appendicitis [22].

12. Acute appendicitis in children

Appendicitis in children is the most common abdominal disease requiring surgery in this age group. The risk of developing appendicitis during a lifetime is reported to be 8.7% for boys and 6.7% for girls. Misdiagnosis rate ranges from 28–57% in 2- to 12-year-old children and approaches to nearly 100% in children younger than 2 years [23].

According to Almaramhy [23], in neonates (birth to 30 days), the most common clinical signs are abdominal distension, vomiting, palpable mass, irritability or lethargy, and cellulitis of the abdominal wall. In infants and toddlers (less than 5 years), the prominent symptoms are vomiting, pain, fever, and diarrhea. Other common symptoms are irritability, cough or rhinitis, grunting respiration, right hip mobility restriction, pain, and limping. On physical examination, a majority of infants (87–100%) have temperature higher than 37°C and diffuse abdominal tenderness (55–92%), whereas localized right lower quadrant tenderness is observed in less than 50% of the cases. Other noticeable signs are lethargy, abdominal distension, rigidity, and abdominal or rectal mass. The delay in the diagnosis most often results in perforation (82–92%) and bowel obstruction (82%).

In order to improve the diagnosis of acute appendicitis in children, two clinical scores have been validated. The Alvarado score (AS) [24] and the Pediatric Appendicitis Score (PAS) [18] were validated in a prospective study by Pogorelic et al. [25] finding that ROC curves gave an area under the curve (AUC) of 0.74 for the AS and 0.73 for the PAS score. They also found a negative appendectomy rate of 14.8% which in the medical literature ranges between 10 and 30%.

In other prospective validation study of the Pediatric Appendicitis score, Goldman et al. [26] found that the PAS score is valid for the diagnosis of acute appendicitis when the score was 7 or greater and for the exclusion of appendicitis when the score was 2 or lower.

In a systematic review, Ebell and Shinholser [27] found that the Alvarado score of 8 or higher rules in the diagnosis of acute appendicitis, whereas one of nine or higher rules in the diagnosis at pretest probabilities greater or equal to 40%. The Pediatric Appendicitis Score did not identify clinically useful low- or high-risk groups at typical pretest probabilities.

Bhatt et al. [28], in a prospective validation of the Pediatric Appendicitis Score in Canada, found that using the ROC curve, the AUC was 0.859. Using a cut point of 5 or less, the score was very sensitive (92.8%) but not very specific (69.3%). They concluded that the PAS is a useful tool in the evaluation of children with possible appendicitis. Scores of 4 or less help rule out appendicitis, while scores of 8 or more help predict appendicitis. Patients with a score of 6–7 may need further evaluation.

Salo et al. [29], in an evaluation of the Pediatric Appendicitis Score in younger and older children, found that younger patients showed a significant inflammation (gangrenous, perforated appendicitis, and appendiceal abscesses) in 75% of cases in comparison to 33.3% in older children. The rate of negative appendectomies was higher among younger children (15.0%) than the older children (6.9%), but not significantly different. Their conclusion was that the PAS scoring system turned out to be a weak tool in diagnosing appendicitis in children, especially in young children.

Yang et al. [30], in a prospective study to evaluate the accuracy of diagnosing appendicitis using the Alvarado score in children, found that from 105 operated patients, 93 (87.6%) were diagnosed with acute appendicitis with an erroneous rate of 12.4%. With an Alvarado score of 6 or greater, the sensitivity and specificity were 86.4 and 80%, respectively. They concluded that the Alvarado score is a noninvasive, safe diagnostic method, which is simple, reliable, and repeatable.

Chisalau et al. [31] conducted a retrospective study in 572 children that underwent surgery for acute appendicitis using the Alvarado score. They found that 16.3% had a negative appendectomy, and that almost all patients with a high score confirmed the diagnosis after surgical intervention. They concluded that the Alvarado score can be a very useful instrument for diagnosing acute appendicitis in early stages of the disease, especially when the score is below 4 or above 8.

Borges et al. [32] carried out a validation study of the Alvarado score in children and teenagers in Brazil. They found that with a cutoff point of 5 or more, a sensitivity of 92.6% and a specificity of 63.0% were obtained. With the same cutoff, the positive predictive value (PPV) was 86.2%, and a negative predictive value was 77.8%. The rate of complicated appendicitis was high it this study. They concluded that the Alvarado score with a cutoff point of 5 or more is a valuable tool in screening children and adolescents for the diagnosis of acute appendicitis.

In an evaluation of the Alvarado score as a diagnostic tool for the diagnosis of appendicitis in children, Heineman and Drake [33] found that a cutoff of 5 appears to be fairly sensitive. They recommended imaging studies on a routine basis for children with a score of 5–7, preferably first ultrasound and only followed by CT scan, if negative, to avoid unnecessary radiation exposure.

Schneider, Kharbanda, and Bachur [34], in a study of 588 children aged 3–21 years, found that the Alvarado score of 7 or greater gave the following results: sensitivity 72%, specificity 81%, PPV 65%, and NPV 85%. This compares with the Samuel score of 6 or greater with the following results: sensitivity 82%, specificity 65%, PPV 58%, and NPV 89%. When the analysis was limited to patients younger than 10 years, the anterior figures did not change dramatically. In this group the area under the curve (AUC) was very similar, 0.83 for the Alvarado score and 0.81 for the Samuel score. In conclusion they found that the Alvarado and Samuel scores provide measurably useful diagnostic information in evaluating children with suspected appendicitis. However, neither method provides sufficiently PPV to be used in clinical practice as a sole method for determination of the need of surgery.

In a systematic review and meta-analysis that included emergency department point-of-care ultrasound (ED-POCUS) and the Pediatric Appendicitis Score (PAS), Benabbas et al. [35] studied two groups of patients: one of "undifferentiated abdominal pain" and another one of "suspected acute appendicitis." In the first group, they included patients with history of pain migration to the right lower quadrant, cough/hop pain, and Rovsing sign pain. For the PAS of 9 or more, the Rovsing sign was the most associated one with acute appendicitis. None of the history, physical examination, laboratory tests, or PAS alone could rule out acute appendicitis in both groups. Using their test-treatment threshold model, positive ED-POCUS could rule in acute appendicitis without the use of CT and MRI, but negative ED-POCUS could not rule out acute appendicitis.

Peyvasteh et al. [36], in a study of 400 children aged less than 12 years, found that anorexia, nausea and vomiting, and rebound tenderness were significantly more common in children with positive appendectomy in contrast to patients with negative appendectomy. Sensitivity and specificity were 91.3 and 38.4%, respectively, and positive predictive value and negative predictive value were 87.7 and 51%, respectively. In children with a modified Alvarado score of more than 7, they found a positive appendectomy of 100% and a negative appendectomy of 15.8%. They concluded that the Modified Alvarado score has high sensitivity but low specificity for diagnosis of acute appendicitis.

13. Acute appendicitis in pregnancy

Acute appendicitis is the commonest non-obstetric surgical emergency during pregnancy, and it may be associated to serious maternal and fetal complications. It occurs in about 1:500–635 pregnancies per year and is more often in the second trimester. Classically, patients describe the appearance of abdominal pain as the first symptom. It begins with periumbilical pain, which then migrates to the right lower quadrant to the extent that the inflammation progresses. Anorexia, nausea, and vomiting, if present, appear after the pain. Fever of up to 38.3°C and leukocytosis may subsequently develop. A pelvic appendix can cause sensitivity below the McBurney's point and other complaints such as an increase in urinary frequency and dysuria or rectal symptoms, such as tenderness, which can confuse the examiner and delay the diagnosis [37]. Microscopic hematuria and leukocyturia may occur when the inflamed appendix is located near the bladder or ureter, but these results are reported in less than 20% of patients. Slight increases in the total serum bilirubin have been described as a marker for perforation of the appendix (70% sensitivity and 86% specificity). C-reactive protein also rises in appendicitis, but it is a nonspecific sign of inflammation. About 80% of nonpregnant patients with appendicitis have preoperative leukocytosis of over 10.000 cells/mL with a left shift. However, mild leukocytosis may be a normal finding in pregnant women in whom the total leukocyte count can reach 16.900 cells in the third trimester, rising to levels around 29.000/mL during labor including slight left shift [37].

Aggenbach et al., in a review of records of 21 pregnant patients suspected of acute appendicitis and subjected to appendectomy, found that 71% had histologically proven appendicitis of whom 43% had non-perforated appendicitis and 29% had perforated appendicitis. The negative appendectomy rate was 29%. The most frequent symptom was pain located in the right lower quadrant (95%). Other common presenting symptoms were nausea (90%), vomiting (48%), and loss of appetite (48%). A classical history of periumbilical pain migrating to the right lower quadrant occurred in 48% of whom two turned out to have a normal appendix. Upon physical examination, right lower quadrant abdominal pain or diffuse abdominal tenderness was seen in the majority of the population, and rebound tenderness was present in 67% of cases. None of the women showed signs of involuntary guarding. Three of 15 women with histologically confirmed appendicitis developed fever (20%). Infection markers such as leukocyte count and C-reactive protein were not significantly raised in pregnant women with appendicitis compared to pregnant women with normal appendix. Of note is that an elevated C-reactive protein (≥10 m/L) was seen in four out of nine pregnant women with non-perforated appendicitis. Three patients with perforated appendicitis generally did not look well. There was no case of fetal demise in this series of 21 patients. In this study, delay in treatment was associated with higher rate of maternal and fetal complications [38].

Tamir et al. found that perforated appendicitis occurred in 43% of patients who had symptoms exceeding 24 hours ($p < 0.0005$). Therefore, establishing the diagnosis of appendicitis accurately and promptly is of utmost importance. The diagnosis of acute appendicitis during pregnancy remains based in upon the combination of history, physical examination, laboratory results, and ultrasonography [39].

Bhandari et al. [40], in a retrospective review of 56 pregnant patients and 164 nonpregnant patients who underwent open appendectomy, reported a negative appendectomy of 21.3% and a perforation rate of 25% in both groups. No maternal or fetal mortality was observed in spite of the high rate of perforation and high rate of complications.

14. Acute appendicitis in the old age

Acute appendicitis, the most common cause of abdominal surgical emergency, shows a different pathogenesis, clinical course, and outcome in the elderly. Age-specific factors are effective on preoperative clinical diagnosis and on the stage of this infectious disease.

Gürleyik G and Gürleyik E studied a series of elderly patients, 50 years of age or older, who were subjected to appendectomy. In a group of 109 older patients, they found that the perforation rate was significantly higher than in pediatric and adult patients. The proportion of the elderly among perforated cases was significantly increased when compared with non-perforated cases (12.9% vs. 2.9%). Postoperative morbidity was noted in 73.8% of perforated and in 11.9% of non-perforated cases with an overall morbidity of 35.9%. The mortality rate was 11.9% in patients with perforation and 1.5% in patients with non-perforated appendicitis. The overall mortality was 5.5%, and no mortality was seen in patients younger than 50 years [41].

Bush et al., in a study of 1.827 adult over 65-year-old patients, who were subjected to open or laparoscopic appendectomy in Swiss hospitals, found that a delay of 12 hours or more was associated with a significant higher frequency of perforated appendicitis (29.7%) than a delay of less than 12 hours. Perforation was associated with higher reintervention rate and increased length of hospital stay [42].

Shchatsko et al., in a retrospective chart review of patients over 65 years old and who were diagnosed with acute appendicitis, found that right lower quadrant tenderness (97.6%), left shift of neutrophils (91.5%), and leukocytosis (84.1%) were the most common symptoms on presentation. This data suggests that altering the interpretation of the Alvarado score to classify elderly patients presenting with a score of 5 or more since a high risk may lead to an earlier diagnosis [43].

Omari et al., in a study of acute appendicitis in the elderly, found that all patients were complaining of abdominal pain. However, the typical migratory pain was described only by 47% of patients, 59% in patients with non-perforated appendix, and 30% in patients with perforated appendix. Anorexia was present in 74% of all patients, but it could not differentiate perforated from non-perforated groups. Nausea and vomiting were present in 57% of patients and were more significantly in the non-perforated group. Of all patients, 41% were febrile at presentation (>38°C), and fever was seen more in the perforated group. Localized tenderness in the right lower abdomen was present in 84% of all patients with 91% in the non-perforated compared with 75% in the perforated group. Although rebound tenderness was found in 75% of the patients, it did not differentiate between both groups. Increased WBC count (>10.000/mm^3) was seen in 63% of all patients at presentation. In the perforated group, 71% of patients had high WBC count associated with 94% shift to the left, compared to 57% patients associated with 61% shift to the left in the non-perforated group. There were six deaths, four in the perforated and two in the nonperforated group [44]. In this study it is interesting to observe that the variables used are exactly the same variables used in the MANTRELS score of Alvarado.

15. Acute appendicitis in developing countries

In developing countries, where there are no facilities to do imaging studies such as abdominal ultrasound or contrast enhanced CT examination in patients suspected of acute appendicitis, the decision to operate depends on clinical grounds.

Madiwa et al., in a retrospective study of black patients in South Africa, showed that appendicitis is twice as common in males as in females and that it occurs predominantly in young people (median age 20 years). The classical presentation of periumbilical pain (16%) was outnumbered by right iliac fossa pain (36%) and nonspecific pain (27%). The majority was perforated (43%), and appendiceal inflammation was the second commonest (37%). The negative appendectomy rate was 8.8%, with a diagnostic error of 14%. Mortality was 2% mainly from patients complicated with peritonitis [45].

Kong et al., in a retrospective study undertaken in South Africa, found that 60% of patients had a perforated appendicitis. Of 599 patients with perforation, 181 (30%) were associated with localized intraabdominal contamination, and the remaining 418 (70%) were associated with generalized intraabdominal sepsis. The median duration from onset of symptoms to first contact with the health care system was 4 days. A third (32%) of patients described a migratory pattern of abdominal pain, and the remaining two thirds (68%) had nonmigratory, nonspecific abdominal pain. Median temperature was 37.5°C; the median heart rate was 101 bpm, and the median leukocyte count was 14,500 cells/mm^3. Other clinical symptoms were nausea/vomiting (79%) and anorexia (58%). They concluded that acute appendicitis in South Africa is a serious disease associated with significant morbidity and with a mortality of 1–2%. Complications associated with appendiceal perforation far exceeded those reported in the developed world. Late presentation is common, with female rural patients suffering the worse clinical outcomes. The cost to the health system is substantial [8].

Abdelahim et al., in a prospective study of adult patients with suspected appendicitis in Sudan, divided these patients in three groups: group 1 with an Alvarado score of 1–3, group 2 with a score of 4–6, and group 3 with a score of 7–10. They found that all patients with an Alvarado score of 7 or above have positive surgical appendicitis. At a cutoff point of 3, the Alvarado score was found to be accurate to rule out acute appendicitis. A negative appendectomy was found in 7.1%, all below 7 of the score, while 37% of patients had a complicated appendectomy with a score of 7 or above [46].

Markar et al. carried out a study to compare management approaches and clinical outcomes of acute appendicitis in Sri Lanka (SL) and the United Kingdom (UK). They found that ultrasound studies were more common in Sri Lanka patients and CT more common in UK patients. More patients underwent open appendectomy in SL group, and laparoscopic approach was utilized more often in the UK group (50.5% vs. 11.9%). Postoperative complications were similarly represented in both groups, but readmissions occurred with greater frequency in the UK group (16.2% vs. 0%). Histological-confirmed appendicitis was seen in a significant proportion of SL patients (93.1% vs. 79.8%). They concluded that methods such as CT do not appear to improve the diagnostic accuracy of appendicitis or prevent complications [47].

Ali and Aliyu, in a retrospective study of 1257 patients, in Nigeria, found a male-to-female ratio of 1:2 and a mean age of 32.4 years. The mean duration of illness was 72 hours. All the patients were admitted with abdominal pain, the majority with pain initially located at the right iliac fossa (38.2%), periumbilical pain (31.3%), and diffused in 27.9%. The most frequent symptoms were: vomiting 85.7%, fever 73.0%, and anorexia 49.9%. Right iliac fossa pain and tenderness were present in 88.46%. The perforation rate was high (23.47%), and the negative appendectomy was 15.9%. Mortality rate was 0.9% [48].

Arfa et al., in a prospective study of 205 patients with acute abdominal pain in the right iliac fossa, found a male-to-female ratio of 0.7:1 and a mean age of 27 years. They classified the patients in three groups: those who had an emergency appendectomy, those who had surgery after an observation period, and those discharged without appendectomy after observation. In the first group of 110 patients, 63% had a rectal temperature greater than 38°C; 44% had guarding of the RIF and 87% elevated white blood counts above 10.000 cells/mm^3. At surgery, appendicitis was diagnosed in 92%. After a mean delay of 36 hours of observation, 50 patients in the second group underwent surgery: 44% had a rectal temperature above 38°C, RIF guarding in 8%, and elevated white blood count above 10.000 cells/mm^3 in 74%. In this group, 94% were diagnosed with appendicitis during surgery. Forty-five patients were discharged without surgery after 36 hours of observation. They concluded that pain and RIF guarding, associated with temperature greater than 38°C, and elevated WBC counts, were predictive of acute appendicitis in 96% of cases. Admission for observation of patients with atypical presentation avoided 45 unnecessary appendectomies [49].

Zognéreh et al., in a retrospective study to analyze clinical, paraclinical, and therapeutic aspects of acute appendicitis in Central Africa Republic, found an incidence of appendectomy in Bangui of 36 per 100,000 inhabitants. These cases of appendicitis were diagnosed essentially on clinical grounds. Leukocyte counts exceeded 10,000 cells/mm^3 in 30% of patients. Histological examination revealed the presence of parasites in 10 cases: *Schistosoma mansoni* eggs, seven cases; *Ascaris lumbricoides* eggs, one case; and combination of these parasites, two cases. Most of patients consulted late, a mean of 4 days, after onset of symptoms. The mortality rate was high, 3.5% partially due to lateness of consultation and because patients in tropical Africa often consult a traditional healer before resorting to modern medicine and also partially from misdiagnosis [50].

Fashima et al., in a prospective study of 250 cases of acute appendicitis in Lagos, Nigeria, found a male-to-female ratio of 1.2:1 with a mean age of 27.7 years and with the majority of cases (42.8%) occurring in the third decade of life. Abdominal pain (100%), fever (48.4%), anorexia (48%), and vomiting (47,8%) were the common symptoms. Commonly elicited signs included right iliac fossa direct tenderness (74.4%), rebound tenderness (59.2%), localized guarding (42.8%), and rectal tenderness (43.2%). The mean white cell count was not significantly elevated (mean 8.538 cell/mm^3). In 63% the appendices were retrocecal with a mean length 10.4 cm. The commonest postoperative complication was wound infection (8%); overall complication rate was 13.5% and a negative appendectomy rate 13.4% [51]. (It is interesting to note the incongruency between the high incidence of rectal tenderness and the high incidence of retrocecal appendices.)

Tade, in Nigeria, carried out a prospective study of 100 consecutive patients who presented to the emergency department with right iliac fossa pain and suspected diagnosis of acute appendicitis. These patients were assessed using the Alvarado score. He found a male-to-female ratio of 1.7:1 and a mean age of 34 years. Of the 100 patients under the study, 38 had appendectomy, and four of these had a normal appendix (19.5%), and seven patients had a perforated appendix (18.4%). Forty-four patients had scores less than 5; they were admitted, and none of them required surgery. Twenty-four patients had appendicitis. The specificity and positive predictive value reached 100% with a score of 10. Sensitivity and negative predictive values reached 100% at scores below 5, indicating that these patients did not have appendicitis [52].

Giiti et al. performed a cross-sectional study in northwest Tanzania, involving 199 patients undergoing appendectomy. In this group they found that 26 patients (13.1%) were HIV-seropositive with a significant older age (mean 38.4 years) than the HIV seronegative population (mean 25.3 years). Leukocytosis was present in 87% of seronegative patients as compared to 34% in seropositive patients. Peritonitis was significantly more frequent among HIV-positives (34% vs. 2%). Also, 11.5% of HIV patients developed surgical site infections, as compared to 0.6% in the HIV-negative group [53].

16. Differential diagnosis in acute appendicitis

In general, when the diagnosis of acute appendicitis is not clear, the clinician has to take into consideration other diagnostic possibilities, and the best form to do it is to assess the patient according to the anatomical location of the pain or tenderness. In this case, the abdomen is divided into four quadrants [54].

If the pain or tenderness is localized in the right upper quadrant, the most probable causes are cholecystitis, biliary colic, cholangitis, hepatitis, hepatic abscess, pancreatitis, peptic ulcer, retrocecal appendicitis, appendicitis during pregnancy, intestinal obstruction, inflammatory bowel disease, and pneumonia.

If the pain is localized in the left upper quadrant, the most probable causes are gastritis, peptic ulcer, pancreatitis, splenomegaly, splenic rupture, intestinal obstruction, inflammatory bowel disease, diverticulitis of the splenic flexure, appendicitis, pneumonia, myocardial ischemia or infarction, and pericarditis.

If the pain is localized in the right lower quadrant, the most probable causes are appendicitis, stump appendicitis, inflammatory bowel disease, diverticulitis (cecal, Merkel's), mesenteric adenitis, intestinal obstruction, hernia, ectopic pregnancy, salpingitis, ovarian cyst, mittelschmerz, nephrolithiasis, pyelonephritis, and ureteral calculus.

If the pain is localized in the left lower quadrant, the most probable causes are colon diverticulitis, appendicitis, intestinal obstruction, inflammatory bowel disease, ischemic colitis, hernia, ectopic pregnancy, salpingitis, ovarian torsion, ruptured ovarian cyst, mittelschmerz, nephrolithiasis, pyelonephritis, and ureteral calculus.

Other probable causes of abdominal pain or tenderness are pneumonia, myocardial ischemia or infarction, pericarditis, gastritis, peptic ulcer, enteritis, colitis, mesenteric thrombosis or ischemia, ruptured abdominal aorta or aneurism, typhoid enteritis, abdominal tuberculosis, parasitic infections, cystitis, epiploic appendagitis, intussusception of the appendix, abdominal cystic lymphangioma, dengue fever, localized pseudomembranous colitis, hemorrhagic omental torsion, and herpes zoster (initial stage).

17. Effect of time on risk of perforation in acute appendicitis

Papaziogas et al. carried out a study to quantify the role of time between symptoms' onset and surgery on the changing risk of appendicitis perforation and to evaluate the possible factors leading to the operation. The relative risk of perforation was calculated according to the "timetable method." Time was divided into intervals, initially 12 hours and, later on, 24 hours. They found that 18 of 169 patients had perforated appendicitis. The time from symptom onset to the first examination was longer for patients with perforation than without ($p = 0.047$). On the other hand, the time from initial examination in the emergency department to the operating room showed no statistical difference between patients with rupture and those without. The risk of perforation was negligible within the first 12 hours of untreated symptoms but increased to 8% within the first 24 hours. Their conclusion was that surgeons should be mindful of delaying surgery beyond 24 hours of symptom onset in patients with assumed appendicitis [55].

Bickell et al. found that for patients with untreated symptoms beyond 36 hours, the risk of rupture rose to and remained steady at 5% for each ensuing period of 12 hours. They also found that patients sent for CT scan experienced longer times to operation (18.6 vs. 7.1 hours) [56].

Andersson mentioned that many studies have shown an association with higher proportion of negative appendectomies in patients with short delay. Early identification and treatment of perforated appendicitis is therefore important. In patients with equivocal diagnosis, active observation is a time-proven, safe, and simple management which gives an improved diagnostic accuracy [57].

18. Basic laboratory tests

The basic laboratory tests that are needed in the early diagnosis of acute appendicitis are just a few. These tests are available in the majority of the health facilities and do not take too much time to obtain the results. They are complete blood count (CBC) that includes a white blood count (WBC) with a differential count. The WBC is a good inflammatory marker that measures the quantitative changes of an inflammatory process and usually run parallel with the increasing temperature. The urinalysis determines if there is excessive number of red cells that could be related to an episode of ureteral calculus. It also may show acetonuria which may be related to anorexia and fasting state. In women of childbearing age, a pregnancy test used is in order to rule out pregnancy. C-reactive protein (CRP) can be used in the late stages of acute appendicitis to confirm complicated appendicitis such as gangrene or perforation of the appendix.

19. Imaging studies

Under certain circumstances, imaging studies may be needed to achieve a correct diagnosis. Sometimes, the clinical presentation of the symptoms is atypical, and the signs and laboratory tests are inconclusive in the diagnosis of acute appendicitis, and in these cases, some imaging studies could be helpful.

Diagnosis of acute appendicitis is usually clinical and straightforward, and extensive investigations are unnecessary. However, a plain X-ray of the abdomen may help in the diagnosis particularly in young children, women of childbearing age, the elderly, and patients with systematic disease or who are immunosuppressed, in whom negative appendectomy and perforation rates are high [58].

The role of plain radiographs in the diagnosis of acute appendicitis has been reviewed in different studies. Many findings have been taken as evidence of appendiceal inflammation, including the presence of a fecalith, dilated sentinel loop of the ileum, ileal or cecal air-fluid levels on the erect film, widened preperitoneal fat line, haziness in the right lower quadrant, and blurring of the right psoas outline. Although plain radiographic findings on the erect or supine plain abdominal films may have an ancillary role in the diagnosis of acute appendicitis, they are neither sufficiently sensitive nor specific. Despite this, the role of plain abdominal radiographs will not become obsolete given the pragmatic difficulties in getting a CT scan as a first-line image and the risk of much greater radiation dose that a CT scan carries [59].

Aydin et al. found that plain abdominal X-ray in children provides useful information in the diagnosis of acute appendicitis and concluded that this test is an important tool not just for exclusion of other causes of pain but also for detection of appendicitis. Careful assessment of plain abdominal films in suspected appendicitis is encouraged in the case of unavailability out of hours of more widely accepted modalities (US, CT). In some cases, unnecessary delay of surgical intervention with a poor outcome may be prevented [60].

Petroianu et al. described the association and relevance of the image of fecal loading in the cecum, detected by plain abdominal X-ray, in patients with acute appendicitis. They studied 170 patients of both sexes who were admitted to the hospital with acute pain in the right flank. One group had plain abdominal X-rays done before surgical treatment, and another group had abdominal plain X-rays done before the surgical procedure and also the following day. They found that the radiographic sign of fecal loading in the cecum of patients with abdominal pain is associated with acute appendicitis. The image usually becomes undetectable shortly after appendix removal. The radiographic sign was present in all pediatric patients, including a 5-day-old premature newborn with perforated appendicitis. Only five of 170 patients without the radiographic sign presented acute appendicitis. This sign strongly supports the diagnosis of acute appendicitis when associated with indicative physical examination and laboratory findings [61].

20. Ultrasound studies

Acute appendicitis remains a clinical diagnosis, but when this diagnosis is uncertain, ultrasound (US) has been proven to be a helpful imaging modality in patient evaluation especially in children with suspicion of appendicitis. Graded compression US is the least expensive and less invasive method and has been reported to have an accuracy of 70–95%.

Toprak et al., in a study to investigate the integration of ultrasound (US) findings with the Alvarado score in diagnosing or excluding acute appendicitis, found that the diagnostic accuracy of US was as follows: sensitivity 93.1%, specificity 92.2%, positive predictive value 92.6%, negative predictive value 93.6%, and accuracy 92.6%. They also found that all patients with an Alvarado score greater than or equal to 7 had appendicitis proven by surgery and pathology. In the case of non-visualization of the appendix without a high Alvarado score, appendicitis can safely be ruled out. CT scan may be useful in children with moderate scores and equivocal findings [62].

The problem with ultrasound is that it was found to have an extremely variable accuracy in the diagnosis of acute appendicitis with a sensitivity range from 44 to 100% and a specificity range of 47 to 99%. Radiologist-operated ultrasound had inferior sensitivity and inferior positive predictive values when compared with a CT scan, though it was significant faster to perform and avoided the administration of contrast materials [63]. For this reason, "a first pass" approach using US first and then CT, if US is not diagnostic, would be desirable in some institutions [64–66]. Chiang found that clinical evaluation is still paramount to the management of patients with suspected acute appendicitis before considering medical imaging like ultrasonography or computed tomography [67]. Nevertheless, in cases of clinical doubt, ultrasonography may improve the diagnosis and reduce the negative laparotomy rate and can also be helpful in detecting periappendicular abscesses or gynecological diseases [68].

21. Computed tomography

In recent years, the routine use of computed tomography in the diagnosis of acute appendicitis has been highly controversial due to concerns related to the hazards of ionizing radiation and also about its overutilization in clear-cut clinical presentations. The use of CT scans of the abdomen exposes the patients to high dose of radiation which may be the equivalent of 400 chest X-rays, and this certainly will increase the risk for development of cancer or leukemia [69–71]. In a prospective randomized study of clinical assessment versus computed tomography for the diagnosis of acute appendicitis, Hong et al. found that clinical assessment, unaided by CT scan, reliably identify patients who needed operation for acute appendicitis, and they undergo surgery sooner, so the routine use of abdominal-pelvic CT is not warranted and computed tomography should not be considered the standard of care for the diagnosis of acute appendicitis [72].

Petrosian found that the overall negative appendectomy rate in patients with CT scan was similar to that in those without (6% for both groups) and that therefore preoperative CT scans did not decrease the negative appendectomy rate [73]. In another study, Lee found that neither CT nor US improves the diagnostic accuracy or the negative appendectomy rate; in fact, they may delay surgical consultation and appendectomy [74]. Using the Alvarado score to decide the need to perform a CT scan in cases of suspected acute appendicitis in the ED settings, McKay found that with a score of 4 to 6, an adjunctive CT scan would be recommended to confirm the diagnosis. If the Alvarado score is 7 or higher, a surgical consultation should be obtained. A computed tomography would be necessary in patients with an Alvarado score of 3 or lower [75]. In another study to compare the Alvarado and CT scan in the evaluation of suspected appendicitis, Tan revealed that CT scans are unnecessary in those patients with an AS of 9 or 10 and recommended that an evaluation by CT scan is of value mainly in patients with an Alvarado score of 6 or less in males and 8 or less in females [76].

22. Magnetic resonance imaging

In a systematic review and meta-analysis of diagnostic performance of MRI for evaluation of acute appendicitis, Duke et al. found that this test has a high accuracy for the diagnosis for a wide range of patients and may be acceptable for use as first-line diagnostic test [77].

Inci et al., in a study to assess the diagnostic value of unenhanced magnetic resonance imaging (MRI) in the diagnosis of acute appendicitis and compare with Alvarado scores and histological results, found that MRI is a valuable technique for detecting acute appendicitis even in the cases with low Alvarado scores [78].

Konrad et al. found that the sensitivity and specificity of MRI for acute appendicitis were 100 and 98%, respectively, as compared to 18 and 99%, respectively, with US. They suggested that at certain institutions, MRI may be considered a first-line imaging modality for pregnant patients of any gestational age with suspected appendicitis [79].

In a retrospective study designed to determine the utility of appendix MRI in evaluation of pediatric patients with right lower quadrant pain and inconclusive appendix sonography findings, Herliczek et al. found that the sensitivity and specificity of MRI for acute appendicitis in children with inconclusive findings were 100 and 96%, respectively. The positive predictive value for the examination was 83%, the negative predictive value was 100%, and the overall test accuracy was 97%. This proves that MRI may supplant CT as a secondary modality to follow inconclusive appendix sonography [80].

In relation to the safety of the use of MRI during the first trimester of pregnancy, Ray et al. found that there is no increased risk of harm to the fetus or to young children. However, Gadolinium-enhanced MRI in pregnancy was associated with increased risk of a broad set of rheumatological, inflammatory, or infiltrative skin conditions from birth and also for stillbirth or neonatal death [81].

23. Diagnostic laparoscopy

Diagnostic laparoscopy for suspected appendicitis is recommended for young women, the elderly, or other patients with unclear pathology because of its broader diagnostic ability and for obese patients due technical difficulties during open laparotomy. In one study the Alvarado score combined with selective laparoscopy gave a rate of 0% cases of negative appendectomy so this approach was recommended for widespread use in the management of suspected acute appendicitis [82].

The difficulty with laparoscopy for the diagnosis of acute appendicitis is that the negative appendectomy rate is higher than open appendectomy because of the absence of tactile feedback. Kraemer et al. found that the negative rates were 22% for laparoscopic appendectomy and 15% for open appendectomy. The role of diagnostic laparoscopy may be useful in a particular subgroup of patients but is not a substitute for good clinical judgment. Furthermore, it is not always necessary to perform an incidental appendectomy [83]. This statement is in conflict with the conclusion of Greason et al. who advised that incidental laparoscopic appendectomy is the preferred treatment option [84].

Strong et al. [85], in a multicenter study, suggested that surgeon's judgment of the intraoperative macroscopic appearance of the appendix is inaccurate and does not improve with seniority and therefore supports removal at the time of surgery. In this study 3326 patients underwent an appendectomy. Documentation of the histopathological specimen was missing in 134 cases, and 34 had no surgeon opinion recorded, leaving 3138 patients for final analysis. Of these patients, 60.5% underwent totally laparoscopic procedures, 32.6% open procedures and 7.0% laparoscopic converted laparoscopic procedures. The authors found that when surgeons assessed an appendix as normal (n = 496), subsequent histological assessment revealed pathology in 138 cases (27.8%). This included 114 patients with appendicitis and 24 patients with other diagnoses (11 worm infestations, five fibrous infiltrations, four carcinoid tumors, two cases of pelvic inflammatory disease within the appendix, one colorectal polyp, and one cecal diverticulum affecting the appendix). On the other hand, where the appendix was judged to be inflamed intraoperatively (n = 2642), pathological assessment revealed a normal appendix in 254 (9.6%). There was overall disagreement in 392 cases (12.5%), leading to only moderate agreement (Kappa 0.571).

Diagnostic laparoscopy and appendectomy for children with chronic right iliac fossa pain have been studied by Charlesworth and Mahomed. Their conclusion was that the literature supports laparoscopic appendectomy in all patients presenting with chronic right iliac fossa pain following negative radiological and serological investigations. Symptomatic improvement can be expected to be 88% immediately and up to 100% in the long term. However, in their study five normal appendices were removed out of 16 children that were subjected to diagnostic laparoscopy and appendectomy [86]. I think that in these cases, it could be a good idea to remove the distal third of the appendix and send it for a frozen section for histological examination during the procedure. In such a way, some of these cases could be spared from a negative appendectomy.

http://dx.doi.org/10.5772/intechopen.75530

24. Unusual cases of acute appendicitis

24.1. Retrocecal appendix

Several unusual cases of acute appendicitis have been found in the medical literature mostly related to abnormal position of the appendix and ethnic variations. Although there is no significant association between retrocecal appendix and perforation [87–89], several cases of serious complications of retrocecal appendicitis have been reported.

Kim et al. [90] described the clinical presentation and computed tomographic features of ascending retrocecal appendicitis. The patients presented with right lower quadrant pain (49%), right flank pain (24%), right upper abdominal pain (18%), and periumbilical pain (15%). Inflamed ascending retrocecal appendices were visualized completely in 70%, partially in 21%, and not detected in 9%. Perforation of the appendix with formation of an abscess was present in 49%, and appendicoliths were found in 33%.

Ong et al. [91] from Singapore reported four cases of patients with retrocecal appendicitis who presented with right upper quadrant abdominal pain. Ultrasound examination showed subhepatic collections in two patients and normal findings in the other two. Computed tomography identified correctly retrocecal appendicitis and inflammation in the retroperitoneum in all cases. In addition, abscesses in the retrocecal space (two cases) and subhepatic collections (two cases) were also demonstrated. Emergency appendectomy was performed in two patients, interval appendectomy in one, and hemicolectomy in another. Surgical findings confirmed the presence of appendicitis and its retroperitoneal extensions.

A case of retroperitoneal necrotizing soft tissue infection after appendicitis was reported by Carmignani et al. [92] where a 17-year-old boy presented to the hospital in acute septic shock after 9 days with symptoms of back pain, fever, and decrease appetite. According to the patient's mother, his pain was originally attributed to chiropractic problems which contributed to the delayed diagnosis. The patient had an acute abdomen and was immediately taken to the operating room for an exploratory laparotomy which revealed an inflamed and perforated retrocecal appendix with diffuse retroperitoneal necrotizing soft tissue infection. An appendectomy was performed, and the patient was resuscitated, stabilized, and transferred to the ICU the same evening. After stabilization the patient was taken to the operating room again for an exploratory laparotomy. At exploration, wide spread necrotizing infection was found involving the anterior abdominal wall, retroperitoneum, and scrotum. Extensive debridement was performed. Subsequently, he remained for utmost 3 months in the hospital for closure of his abdominal wound by plastic surgery team. This initially required debridement with placement of a xenograft and a foam, polyethylene, dressing. The patient's abdominal wound was later closed with a split-thickness graft. The patient's condition continued to progress satisfactorily, and he was discharged.

One case of acute appendicitis mimicking acute scrotum was reported by Buzatti et al. [93] in a young male who presented with diffuse abdominal pain of 4-day duration, accompanied by fever and anorexia. On physical examination the scrotum was red and swollen, and there was tenderness by direct percussion of the lower abdomen. The skin around the scrotum, mainly in the groin and hypogastric area, was also red suggesting evolution of a Fournier syndrome. A white blood cell count was elevated (18.000 cells/mm^3), and C-reactive protein was about 260. Intensive care support and antibiotic therapy were immediately started. An ultrasonography of the scrotum was performed, which showed the vascularization of both testicles preserved, and an abscess in the right hemiscrotum and the presence of edema in the subcutaneous and the muscular fascia of the abdominal wall and inguinal region. An abdominal ultrasound demonstrated free liquid in the pelvis but did not find the appendix. The scrotal abscess was drained, and the left hemiscrotum cavity was also explored finding no pus or necrosis inside. Afterward a laparotomy was performed and a retrocecal appendix was found with diffuse peritonitis. Appendectomy was performed followed by abdominal cavity wash. The patient developed infectious complications and survived. Pathological examination confirmed an acute perforated appendicitis.

Hsieh et al. [94] reported two cases of retroperitoneal abscess resulting from perforated acute appendicitis and identified 22 more cases. In this series, they found that none of the patients presented with classical symptoms of acute appendicitis at the onset of the disease and less than half reported abdominal pain. The average interval between the onset of symptoms and diagnosis was 16 days, and the most effective tool was computed tomography. The mortality rate was 16.7%, and all deaths were caused by profound sepsis.

Sharma [95] described a case of retrocecal appendicitis in a 6-year-old boy who presented with a thigh abscess. He presented with a positive psoas sign and feculent discharge in the right thigh. Laparotomy revealed a perforated retrocecal appendix with surrounding collection communicating to the thigh. Appendectomy with drainage of the retroperitoneal and thigh collections under adequate antibiotic coverage resulted in a satisfactory recovery.

24.2. Stump appendicitis

Stump appendicitis is defined as the development of obstruction and inflammation of the residual appendix after appendectomy. In a 60-year literature review of stump appendicitis, Subramanian and Liang [96] found that stump appendicitis is an underreported and poorly defined condition. Their conclusion was that appendicitis warrants early detection in patients with abdominal pain, nausea, and vomiting. A prior history of appendectomy can delay the diagnosis which could lead to perforation that requires extensive resection.

Roberts et al. [97] identified 48 cases of stump appendicitis in the English medical literature and found that the presenting symptoms are basically indistinguishable from those of primary appendicitis. They found three cases of stump appendicitis in their institution that were diagnosed ranging from 2 months to 20 years after the initial appendectomy. In their review, they found perforation of the appendix in 60% of patients. Besides the possibility of stump appendicitis, there is the possibility of a duplicate appendix which is a rare developmental abnormality. In the review of these 48 cases, one can see that there is a difference among the length of the stumps removed. The average length of the stumps left after the initial operation was 2.7 cm for an open appendectomy vs. 4.2 cm for a laparoscopic appendectomy which indicates that there is certain difficulty to identify the cecal appendiceal junction during the laparoscopic appendectomy.

Geraci et al. [98] reported a case of a 54-year-old appendicectomized woman who presented with a recent history of periumbilical abdominal pain radiating to the right side and right iliac fossa, in the absence of fever, vomiting, or other symptoms. Elective colonoscopy revealed an appendicular orifice clogged by a big fecalith with surrounding hyperemic mucosa. A CT scan confirmed the diagnosis of stump appendicitis. After 30 days of therapy with metronidazole and mesalazine, the patient was submitted to surgery and appendectomy was performed obtaining a specimen of 24 mm stump appendicitis.

Bu-Ali et al. [99] reported a case of stump appendicitis after laparoscopic appendectomy which was diagnosed preoperatively with a CT scan. This case was of an 18-year-old male who presented with a 1-week history of lower abdominal pain, nausea, and vomiting. He had a history of laparoscopic appendectomy for acute appendicitis. On physical examination, he had tenderness and guarding in the lower abdomen. A CT scan showed free pelvic fluid with a tubular structure of about 2.5 cm in length and 0.78 cm in diameter located posteriorly to the ileocecal junction. Laparoscopic exploration confirmed the findings. A residual appendicular stump was found and dissected from adhesions and removed. Histopathology showed a residual appendix with residual neutrophilic infiltration associated with multifocal hemorrhagic necrosis. The postoperative was uneventful.

Tang et al. [100] reported three cases of stump appendicitis in children who presented with right lower quadrant abdominal pain and a history of appendectomy. Ramirez et al. [101] reported a case of stump appendicitis in a 2-year-old child admitted to the emergency room due to vomiting, abdominal pain, and fever. The patient had a history of peritonitis associated with perforated appendicitis 6 months before. At this time, he had an emergency laparotomy due to hemodynamic deterioration and worsening of abdominal pain. During the operation, peritonitis, stump appendicitis with perforation, and incidental Meckel's diverticulum was found. This required removal of the stump and the Meckel's diverticulum and intestinal resection with an end-to-end anastomosis. Patient received antibiotic therapy and underwent a laparostomy with subsequent peritoneal lavages in the ICU. He was discharged in good general condition 14 days after surgery.

24.3. Left-sided appendicitis

Congenital anatomical abnormalities resulting in left-sided appendicitis are usually caused by situs inversus and midgut malrotation. Several cases have been reported in different parts of the world, some of them starting with diffused abdominal pain and then localizing into the left upper quadrant or in the left lower quadrant. Akbulut et al. [102] gave an overview of the literature on left-sided appendicitis associated with situs inversus totalis and midgut malrotation. They found that the diagnosis was made preoperatively in 51.5% of the cases and intraoperatively in 19% of cases. Pain location was present in the left lower quadrant in 62% of cases, right lower quadrant (14.7%), bilateral lower quadrant (7.3%), pelvic region (2%), left upper quadrant (7.3%), and periumbilical area (6.3%).

Singla et al. [103] reported a case of left-sided acute appendicitis in an elderly male with asymptomatic midgut rotation. Their conclusion was that imaging offers significant advantage for timely and definitive management.

24.4. Abdominal wall hernias and acute appendicitis

Amyand's hernia is a rare form of an inguinal hernia (less than 1% inguinal hernias) which occurs when the appendix is included in the hernia sac and becomes incarcerated. Claudius Amyand was a French surgeon who performed the first successful appendectomy in 1735. He found a perforated appendix with a pin within an inguinal hernia sac, and since then a few similar cases have been reported in the medical literature. Perforated appendix and periappendicular abscess formation within an inguinal sac is an extremely rare condition.

Unver et al. [104] presented a case of left-sided Amyand's hernia in which a 32-year-old male presented with an irreducible inguinal mass with pain for 3 days accompanied by nausea and vomiting. He had a Lichtenstein hernioplasty 3 years before for a left inguinal hernia. An abdominal CT scan showed a mobile cecum that switched to the left side of the abdomen, with coexisting inflammatory echogenic findings and a left-sided inguinal hernia sac including an appendix vermiformis. The patient underwent an emergency abdominal exploration finding that the cecum was mobile and shifted to the left side. The appendix was found incarcerated in the left inguinal sac. The appendix was removed, and the internal ring was repaired with primary sutures.

The presence of an appendix within a femoral hernia sac is a rare condition and is known as a De Garengeot hernia, after a French surgeon who first described it in the literature in 1731. This type of hernia is reported to account for 0.5–3.3% of all femoral hernias.

Ebisawa et al. [105] reported a case of De Garengeot hernia in which a 90-year-old female presented with a 3-day history of right inguinal swelling and inguinal pain. On physical examination there was an egg-sized mass located slightly lower than the inguinal ligament that showed signs of inflammation and was painful on direct compression. There were no complaints of abdominal pain, nausea, or vomiting. Laboratory tests revealed a slight elevation of CRP (0.49 mg/dL). Abdominal X-ray showed no gas-fluid levels and no signs of small intestine dilatation. Pelvic CT scan revealed a small round mass beside the femoral artery and vein with air-fluid levels and small amount of ascites in the pelvic cavity. The patient was taken to the operating room, and the inguinal ligament was transected. The hernial sac revealed a congested and inflamed appendix. Appendectomy was performed through the hernial sac. There was no evidence of perforation or abscess, so a hernioplasty was completed with synthetic mesh. Histopathological examination revealed a gangrenous appendicitis. The patient was discharged 7 days later with no complications. Because of the rarity and lack of typical symptoms associated with acute appendicitis, achieving preoperative diagnosis is very difficult.

25. Conclusion

Diagnosis of acute appendicitis is basically made on clinical grounds where the experience and common sense of the physician are extremely important. The main purpose of this approach is to make a timely and accurate diagnosis within the first 24 hours after the initiation of symptoms in order to prevent serious complications such as gangrene and perforation of the appendix.

Author details

Alfredo Alvarado[1,2,3,4,5]*

*Address all correspondence to: alfredoalvara@hotmail.com

1 Alma mater: Universidad Nacional de Colombia, Bogotá, Colombia

2 Certified by the American Board of Surgery and the American Board of Emergency Medicine, Miami, FL, USA

3 International College of Surgeons, Chicago, IL, USA

4 Society of Laparoscopic Surgeons, Chicago, USA

5 American College of Emergency Physicians, Irving TX, USA

References

[1] Craig S, Brenner BE. Appendicitis: Practice essentials, backgrounds, anatomy. Medscape. Jan 19, 2017

[2] Buckius MT, McGrath B, Monk J, Grim R, Bell T, Ahuja V. Journal of Surgical Research. 2012;**175**:185-190

[3] Wagensteen OH, Dennis C. Experimental proof of the obstructive origin of appendicitis in man. Annals of Surgery. 1939;**110**:629-647

[4] Singh JP, Mariadson JG. Role of the fecalith in modern-day appendicitis. Annals of the Royal College of Surgeons of England. 2013 Jan;**95**(1):48-51

[5] Peterson MC, Holbrook JH, Von Hales D, Smith NL, Stacker LV. Contributions of the history, physical examination, and laboratory investigation. The Western Journal of Medicine. 1992 Feb;**156**(2):163-165

[6] Graff L, Russel J, Seashore J, et al. False-negative and false- positive errors in abdominal pain evaluation: Failure to diagnose acute appendicitis and unnecessary surgery. Academic Emergency Medicine. 2000 Nov;**7**(11)

[7] Sedlack JD. The rising morbidity of appendectomy for acute appendicitis. Welcome to Appendicitis.pro.Google (direct Web citation)

[8] Kong VY, Sartorius B, Clarke DL. Acute appendicitis in the developing world is a morbid disease. Annals of the Royal College of Surgeons of England. 2015;**00**:1-6

[9] Cope Z. The Early Diagnosis of the Acute Abdomen. Ely House, London: Oxford University Press; 1968

[10] Wagner J, McKinney WP, Carpenter JL. Does this adult patient have appendicitis? The rational clinical examination. American Medical Association. Chapter 5. 2009. p. 54

[11] Gauderer MW, Crane MM, Green HA, Decou JM, Abrams RS. Acute appendicitis in children: The importance of family history. Journal of Pediatric Surgery. 2001 Aug;**36**(8): 1214-1217

[12] Ergul E. Importance of family history and genetics for the prediction of acute appendicitis. The Internet Journal of Surgery. 2006;**10**(1)

[13] Shperber Y, Halevy A, Oland J, Orda R. Familial retrocecal appendicitis. Journal of the Royal Society of Medicine. 1966 Jul;**79**:405-406

[14] Alary FS, Gutierrez I, Perez JG. Familial history aggregation on acute appendicitis. BMJ Case Reports. 19 Oct, 2017. p. 1-3

[15] Humes DH, Simpson J. Clinical presentation of acute appendicitis: Clinical signs, laboratory findings, clinical scores, Alvarado score and derivative scores. Imaging of Acute Appendicitis in Adults and Children. Medical Radiology. Springer-Verlag Berlin Heidelberger; 2011

[16] Ying-Lie O. Contribution of Clinical Features in Appendicitis Scores: An International Systematic Review. Albinusdreef 2, 2333 ZA Leiden, Netherlands: Leiden University Medical Center. Jan 2012

[17] Petroianu A. Diagnosis of acute appendicitis. International Journal of Surgery. 2012;**10**: 115-119

[18] Samuel M. Pediatric appendicitis score. Journal of Pediatric Surgery. 2002;**37**:877-881

[19] Markle GB. A simple test for intraperitoneal inflammation. The American Journal of Surgery. 1973;**125**:721

[20] Massouh sign. Wikipedia (Published Online)

[21] Wani I. K-sign in retrocecal appendicitis: A case review series. Cases Journal. 2009;**2**:157 (Published Online)

[22] Hambuger sign. Wikipedia (Published Online)

[23] Almaramhy HH. Acute appendicitis in young children less than 5 years: Review article. Italian Journal of Pediatrics. 2017;**43**:15

[24] Alvarado A. A practical score for the early diagnosis of acute appendicitis. Annals of Emergency Medicine. 1986;**15**(5):557-564

[25] Pogorelic Z, Rak S, Mrklic I, Juric I. Prospective validation of Alvarado score and pediatric appendicitis score for the diagnosis of acute appendicitis in children. Pediatric Emergency Care. 2015;**31**:164-168

[26] Goldman RD, Carter S, Stephen D, Antoon R, Mounstephen W, Langer JC. Prospective validation of the pediatric appendicitis score. The Journal of Pediatrics. 2008;**153**:278-282

[27] Ebell MH, Shinholser JA. What are the most clinically useful cutoffs for the Alvarado and pediatric appendicitis scores? A systematic review. Annals of Emergency Medicine. 2014 Oct;**64**(4):365-362

[28] Bhatt M, Joseph L, Ducharme FM, Dougherty G. Prospective validation of the pediatric appendicitis score in Canadian pediatric emergency department. Academic Emergency Medicine. 2009 Jul;**16**(7):591-596

[29] Salo M, Friman G, Stenstrom P, Ohlson B, Arnbjonson E. Appendicitis in children: Evaluation of the pediatric appendicitis score in younger and older children. Surgery Research and Practice, Hindawi Publishing Corporation; 2014:6. Article: 438076

[30] Yang ES, Yoon SK, Kim EY, Rho YI, Park SK, Moon KR. Usefulness of Alvarado scoring system for the diagnosis of acute appendicitis in children. Korean Journal of Pediatric Gastroenterology and Nutrition. 2004 Mar;**7**(1):1-7

[31] Chisalau V, Tica C, Chirila S, Ionescu C. ARS Medical Tomitana. 2017;**3**(23):115-129

[32] Borges PS, Lima M, Falbo Neto GH. The Alvarado score validation in diagnosing acute appendicitis in children and teenagers at the Instituto Materno Infantil de Pernambuco. Rev Bras Saude Mater infant. 2003;**3**(4):439-445

[33] Heineman J. Am evaluation of the Alvarado score as a diagnostic tool for appendicitis in children. BestBets. April 2013 (Published Online)

[34] Schneider C, Kharbanda A, Bachur R. Evaluating appendicitis scoring systems using prospective pediatric cohort. Annals of Emergency Medicine. 2007 Jun;**49**(6):778-784

[35] Benabbas R, Hanna M, Shah J, Sinert R. Diagnostic accuracy of history, physical examination, laboratory tests, and point of care ultrasound for pediatric acute appendicitis in the emergency department: A systematic review and meta-analysis. Academic Emergency Medicine. 2017;**24**(5):523-551

[36] Peyvasteh M, Askarpour S, Javaherizadeh H, Besharati S. Modified Alvarado score in children with diagnosis of appendicitis. Arquivos Brasileiros de Cirurgia Digestiva. 2017; **30**(1):51-52

[37] Franca-Neto AH, do Amorin MM, Virgolino-Nobrega BMS. Acute appendicitis in pregnancy: Literature review. Revista Da Associacao Medica Brasileira. 2015 Mac/Apr;**61**(2): 1-14

[38] Aggenbach L, Zeeman GG, Cantineau AEP, et al. Impact of appendicitis during pregnancy: No delay in accurate diagnosis and treatment. International Journal of Surgery. 2015;**15**:84-89

[39] Tamir IL, Bongard FS, Klein SR. Acute appendicitis in the pregnant patient. The American Journal of Surgery. 1990 Dec;**160**(6):571-575

[40] Bhandari TR, Shahi S, Acharya S. Acute appendicitis in the developing world. International Scholarly Research Notices. 2017;**2017**:2636759

[41] Gurleyik G, Gurleyik E. Age related clinical features in older patients with acute appendicitis. European Journal of Emergency Medicine. 2003 Sep;**10**(3):200-203

[42] Busch M, Gutzwiller FS, Aellig S, et al. In-hospital delay increases the risk of perforationin adults with acute appendicitis. World Journal of Surgery. 2011 Jul;**35**(7):1626-1633

[43] Shchatsko A, Brown R, Reid T, et al. The utility of the Alvarado score in the diagnosis of acute appendicitis in the elderly. The American Journal of Surgery. 2017 July;**83**(7):793-798

[44] Omari AH, Khammash MR, Qasaimeh GR, et al. Acute appendicitis in the elderly: Risks factors of perforation. World Journal of Emergency Surgery;**214, 9**:6

[45] Madiba TE, Haffejee, Mbete DL, et al. Appendicitis among African patients at king Edward VIII hospital, Durban, South Africa: A review. East African Medical Journal. 1998 Feb;**75**(2):81-84

[46] Abdelahim M, Khair R, Elsiddig K. The validity of the Alvarado score in diagnosis of acute appendicitis among Sudanese patients. Surgery: Current Research. 2016;**6**:1

[47] Markar SR, Pinto D, Penna M, et al. A comparative international study on the management of acute appendicitis between a developed country and a middle-income country. International Journal of Surgery. 2014;**12**(4):357-360

[48] Ali N, Aliyu S. Appendicitis and its surgical management experience at the university of Maidiguri teaching hospital Nigeria. Nigerian Journal of Medicine. 2012 Apr-Jun;**21**(2): 223-226

[49] Arfa N, Gharbi L, Marsaoui L, et al. Value of admission for observation in the management of acute abdominal right iliac fossa pain. Prospective study of 205 cases. La Presse Médicale. 2006 Mar;**35**(3):393-398

[50] Zoguereh DD, Lemaitre X, Ikoli JF, et al. Acute appendicitis at the National University Hospital in Bangui, Central African Republic: Epidemiologic, clinical, paraclinical and therapeutic aspects. Sante 2001 Apr-Jun;**11**(2):117-125

[51] Ib F, Adesanya AA, Atoyebi OA, et al. Acute appendicitis in Lagos: A review of 250 cases. The Nigerian Postgraduate Medical Journal. 2009 Dec;**16**(4):268-273

[52] Tade AO. Evaluation of Alvarado score as an admission criterion in patients with suspected diagnosis of acute appendicitis. West African Journal of Medicine. 2007;**26**(3):210-212

[53] Giiti GC, Mazig HD, Heulkelbach H, Mahalu W. HIV, appendectomy and postoperative comlications at a reference hospital in Northwest Tanzania: Cross-sectional study. AIDS Research and Therapy. 2010 Dec 29;**7**:47

[54] Hardy A, Butler B, Crandall M. The evaluation of the acute abdomen. In: Moore LJ et al. editors. Common Problems in Acute Care Surgery. New York; Springer Science+Business Media; 2013

[55] Papaziogas B, Tsiaousis P, Koutelidakis, et al. Effect of time on risk of perforation in acute appendicitis. Acta Chirurgica Belgica. 2009 Jan-Feb;**109**(1):75-80

[56] Bickell NA, Aufses AH, Rojas M, Bodian C. How time affects the risk of rupture in appendicitis. Journal of the American College of Surgeons. 2008 Mar;**202**(3):401-406

[57] Andersson RE. Does delay of diagnosis and treatment in appendicitis cause perforation? World Journal of Surgery. 2016;**40**:1315-1317

[58] Rodrigues G, Kanniayan L, Gopashetty M, et al. Plain X-ray in acute appendicitis. Internet Journal of Radiology. 2003;**3**(2):1-4

[59] Bin Ismail HM, Malik A. Will plain abdominal X-ray become obsolete? Open Journal of Radiology. 2017;**2**(2):32-27

[60] Aydin D, Turan C, Yurtseven A, et al. Integration of radiological findings and a clinical score in pediatric patients. Pediatrics International. 2017 Dec;**60**(2):173-178. DOI: 1111/ped.13471

[61] Petroianu A, Alberti L, Zac RI. Assessment of the persistence of fecal loading in the cecum in presence of acute appendicitis. International Journal of Surgery. 2007;**5**:11-16

[62] Toprak H, Kilinkaslan H, Ahmad IC, et al. Integration of ultrasound findings with Alvarado score in children with suspected appendicitis. Pediatrics International. 2014;**56**:95-99

[63] Pinto F, Pinto A, Russo A, et al. Accuracy of ultrasonography in the diagnosis of acute appendicitis in adult patients: Review ultrasound. Critical Ultrasound Journal. 2013;**5** (Suppl 1):52

[64] Reich B, Zalut T, Weiner S. An international evaluation of ultrasound vs computed tomography in the diagnosis of appendicitis. International Journal of Emergency Medicine. 2011;**4**:68

[65] Mostbeck G, Adam EJ, Nielsen MB, et al. How to diagnose acute appendicitis: Ultrasound first. Insights imaging. 2016 Apr;**7**(2):255-263

[66] Debnath J, George RA, Ravikumar R. Imaging in acute appendicitis: What, when, and why. Medical Journal Armed Forces India. 2017;**73**:74-79

[67] Chiang DT, Tan EI, Birks D. To have or not to have. Should computed tomography and ultrasonography be implemented as a routine in patients with suspected appendicitis in a regional hospital? Annals of the Royal College of Surgeons of England. 2008;**90**:17-21

[68] John H, Neff U, Kelemen N. Appendicitis diagnosis today. Clinical and ultrasound deductions. World Journal of Surgery. 1993;**17**:243-249

[69] Mettler FA et al. Effective doses in radiology and diagnostic nuclear medicine: A catalog. Radiology. 2008;**24**(1):254-263

[70] Guite KM, Hinshaw LH, Ranallo FN, et al. Ionizing radiation in abdominal CT: Unindicated multiphase scans are an important source of medically unnecessary exposure. Journal of the American College of Radiology. 2011;**8**:756-761

[71] Markar SR, Karthikesalingan A, Cunningham J, et al. Increase use of preoperative imaging and laparoscopy has no impact on clinical outcomes in patients undergoing appendectomy. Annals of the Royal College of Surgeons of England. 2011;**93**:620-623

[72] Hong JJ, Cohn SM, Ekeh P, et al. A prospective randomized study of clinical assessment versus computed tomography for the diagnosis of acute appendicitis. Surgical Infections. 2003;**4**(3):231-239

[73] Petrosian M, Estrada J, Chan S, et al. CT scan in patients with suspected appendicitis: Clinical implications for the acute care surgeon. European Surgical Research. 2008;**40**(2): 211-210

[74] Lee SL, Walsh AJ, Ho HS. Computed tomography and ultrasonography do not improve and may delay the diagnosis and treatment of acute appendicitis. Archives of Surgery. 2001;**136**:556-562

[75] McKay R, Shepherd J. The use of the clinical score system by Alvarado in the decision to perform computed tomography for acute appendicitis in the ED. American Journal of Emergency Medicine. 2007;**25**(50):489-493

[76] Tan WJ, Acharyya S, Goh YV, et al. Prospective comparison of the Alvarado score and CT scan in the evaluation of suspected appendicitis: A proposed algorithm to guide CT use. Journal of the American College of Surgeons. 2015;**220**:218-224

[77] Duke E, Kalb B, Arif-Tiwari, et al. A systematic review and meta-analysis of diagnostic performance of MRI for evaluation of acute appendicitis. American Journal of Roentgenology. 2016;**206**(3)

[78] Inci E, Hocauglu E, Aydin S, et al. Efficiency of unenhanced MRI in the diagnosis of acute appendicitis: Comparison with Alvarado scoring system and histopathological results. European Journal of Radiology. 2011;**80**(2):253-258

[79] Konrad J, Grand D, Lourenco A. MRI: First-line imaging modality for pregnant patients with suspected appendicitis. Abdominal Imaging. 2015 Oct;**40**(8):3359-3364

[80] Herliczek TW, Swenson DW, Mayo-Smith WW. Utility of MRI after inconclusive ultrasound in pediatric patients with suspected appendicitis: Retrospective review of 60 consecutive patients. American Journal of Roentgenology. 2013;**200**:968-973

[81] Ray JG, Vermeulen MJ, Bharatha A, et al. Association between MRI exposure during pregnancy and fetal and childhood outcomes. JAMA. 2016 Sep 6;**316**(9):952-961

[82] Borgstein PJ, Gordijn RV, Eijsbouts QA. Cuesta MA. Acute appendicitis, a clear-cut case for men a guessing game in young women. A prospective study on the role of laparoscopy. Surgical Endoscopy. 1997;**11**(9):923-927

[83] Kraemer M, Ohman C, Leoppert R, Yang O. Macroscopic assessment of the appendix at diagnostic laparoscopic is reliable. Surgical Endoscopy. 2000 Jul;**14**(7):625-633

[84] Greason KL, Rappold JG, Liberman MA. Incidental laparoscopic appendectomy for acute right lower quadrant abdominal pain. Its time has come. Surgical Endoscopy. 1998 Mar;**12**(3):223-225

[85] Strong S, Blencowe N, Bhangu A. How good are surgeons at identifying appendicitis? Results from a multi-Centre cohort study. International Journal of Surgery. 2015;**15**:107-112

[86] Charlesworth Charlesworth P, Mahomed A. Diagnostic laparoscopy and appendectomy for children with chronic right iliac fossa pain: An aggregate analysis. Journal of Population and Social Studies:1

[87] Shen GK, Wong R, Daller J, et al. Does the retrocecal position of the vermiform appendix alter the clinical course of acute appendicitis? A prospective analysis. Archives of Surgery. 1991 May;**126**(5):569-570

[88] Herscu G, Kong A, Russell D, et al. Retrocecal appendix location and perforationat presentation. The American Journal of Surgery. 2006 Oct;**72**(10):890-893

[89] Oruc M, Muminagic S, Denjalic A, et al. Retrocaecal appendix position: Findings during the classic appendectomy. Medical Archives. 1912 Jun;**66**(3):190-193

[90] Kim S, Lim HK, Lee JY, et al. Ascending retrocecal appendicitis: Clinical and computed tomographic findings. Journal of Computer Assisted Tomography. 2006 Sep-Oct;**30**(5): 772-776

[91] Ong EMW, Venkatesh K. Ascending retrocecal appendicitis presenting with right upper abdominal pain: Utility of computed tomography. World Journal of Gastroenterology. 2009 Jul 28;**15**(28):3576-3579

[92] Carmignani CP, Ismail S, Ganz J, Kalan MMH. Retroperitoneal necrotizing soft tissue infection after appendicitis. Surgical Rounds. 2005 June:283-284

[93] Buzatti KC, Goncalvez MV, Da Silva R, Rodrigues BP. Acute appendicitis mimicking acute scrotum: A rare complication of a common abdominal inflammatory disease. Journal of Coloproctology. 2018;(1):65-69

[94] Hsieh CH, Wang JC, Yang HR, et al. Retroperitoneal abscess resulting from perforated acute appendicitis: Analysis of its management and outcome. Surgery Today. 2007;**37**:762-767

[95] Sharma SB, Gupta V, Sarma SC. Acute appendicitis presenting as thigh abscess in a child: A case report. Pediatric Surgery International. 2005 Apr;**21**(4):298-300

[96] Subramanian A, Liang MK. A 60-year literature review of stump appendicitis: The need for a critical view. American Journal of Surgery. 2012 Apr;**203**(4):503-507

[97] Roberts KE, Starker LF, Andrew J, et al. Stump appendicitis: a surgeon's dilemma. Journal of the Society of Laparoendoscopic Surgeons. 2011;**15**:373-378

[98] Geraci G, Di Carlo G, Cudia B, Modica G. Stump appendicitis. A case report. International Journal of Surgery Case Reports. 2016;**20**:21-23

[99] Bu-Ali O, Al-Bashir M, Samir HA, Abu-Sidan FM. Stump appendicitis after laparoscopic appendectomy: Case report. Ulusal Travma ve Acil Cerrahi Dergisi. 2011 May;**17**(3):267-268

[100] Tang XB, Qu RB, Wang WL. Stump appendicitis in children. Journal of Pediatric Surgery. 2011;**6**(1):233-236

[101] Ramirez AG, Fierro F, Holguin DA, Mendez M. Stump appendicitis in a 2-year-old patient. Case Report and Literature Review. 2017 Jan;**3**(1)

[102] Akbulut S, Ulku A, Senol A, et al. Left-sided appendicitis: Review of 95 published cases and a case report. World Journal of Gastroenterology. 2010 November 28;**16**(44):5598-5602

[103] Singla A, Rajaratman J, Singla AA. Unusual presentation of left sided appendicitis in elderly male with asymptomatic midgut rotation. International Journal of Surgery Case Reports. 2015;**17**:42-44

[104] Unver M, Ozturk S, Karaman K, Turgut E. Left sided Amyand's hernia. World Journal of Gastrointestinal Surgery. 2013 Oct 27;**5**(10):285-286

[105] Ebisawa K, Yamzaki S, Kimura Y, et al. Acute appendicitis in an incarcerated femoral hernia: A case of De Garendeot hernia. Case Reports in Gastroenterology. 2009 Sep-Dec;**3**(3):313-317

Chapter 3

Diagnostic Scores in Acute Appendicitis

Alfredo Alvarado

Additional information is available at the end of the chapter

http://dx.doi.org/10.5772/intechopen.77230

Abstract

Diagnostic scores should be part of the initial evaluation of patients suspected of acute appendicitis. This approach could be very helpful in order to make an early diagnosis and to stratify the cases for observation, further investigation, or surgical intervention.

Keywords: diagnostic scores in acute appendicitis, Alvarado score, clinical approach

1. Introduction

Several scoring systems have been developed to help clinicians in the diagnosis of acute appendicitis. The best-known scores are the Alvarado score, the modified Alvarado score, the Pediatric Appendicitis Score, the Appendicitis Inflammatory Response score, and the RIPASA score. These tools not only can be used for diagnostic purposes but also for stratification, separating those patients who require observation and workup from those who can be assigned for certain specific treatment. The aim of these scores is to reduce the number of negative appendectomies without increasing the number of perforations.

The Alvarado score was described in 1986 [1] and since then has been evaluated and validated in many studies. It consists of three symptoms, three clinical signs, and two laboratory tests. This system uses a simple mnemonics (**MANTRELS**) that is easy to remember and can be applied in many settings without the need of a computer. The symptoms are migration (one point), anorexia-acetonuria (one point), and nausea/vomiting (one point). The clinical signs are tenderness in the right lower quadrant (two points), rebound pain (one point), and elevation of oral temperature (37.3°C or more) (one Point).

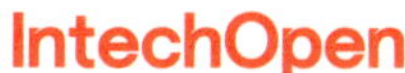

The basic laboratory tests are a complete blood count (CBC) to look for leukocytosis (>10,000 cells/mm^3) and a differential white blood count (WBC) looking for left **shift** (increased stabs >5% or segmented neutrophils >75%). A urinalysis is useful to determine if there is acetone, which indicates the presence of a fasting state related to anorexia, and also, it may show many red cells due to an inflammatory process around the appendix. If the urine shows too many red cells, it may point to a ureteral calculus, and further investigation should be done. The C-reactive protein (CRP) test is not included in the score because it is a nonspecific test that detects an inflammatory process only and is not diagnostic for any particular condition. Besides this, it would be a redundancy since the shift to the left and leukocytosis are doing the same thing. Furthermore, it will not help in the initial stages of acute appendicitis because it will defeat the purpose of the score, that is to say, to make an early diagnosis of acute appendicitis.

Direct tenderness on the right lower quadrant can be replaced by direct percussion with the fist, as a mallet, on the right lumbar area in cases of retrocecal appendicitis which occurs in 75–85% of cases.

Rebound pain can be replaced by other indirect signs such as the Rovsing sign, Dunphy sign (cough test) or the Markle's test (heel-drop jarring test), pain on walking, pain with jolts or bumps in the road, and the inspiration test. Uncommon tests of peritoneal irritation such as the psoas and the obturator tests can replace the rebound pain test also. In children who are unable to communicate well, cutaneous hyperesthesia can be added to replace the migration symptom.

In order of decreasing importance, the best predictive factors proved to be localized tenderness on the right lower quadrant, leukocytosis, migration of pain, shift to the left, temperature elevation, nausea or vomiting, anorexia or acetone in the urine, and direct rebound pain. Two points are assigned to the more important factors (tenderness and leukocytosis) and a value of 1 for each one of the others, for a possible total score of 10. A score of 4–5 is compatible with the diagnosis of acute appendicitis, a score of 7 or 8 indicates a probable appendicitis, and a score of 9 or 10 indicates a very probable appendicitis. To this score the clinician could subtract two points if the patient complains of headache because this symptom is very rare in cases of acute appendicitis. In this particular situation, the patient may need further investigation to rule out a different disorder.

Scores of 5 or 6 are in a gray area, and in this case, the clinician may want to observe the patient for a short time (reevaluate every 4–6 hours) for 12–24 hours, and if the score remains, the same consider other tests such as ultrasound or diagnostic laparoscopy. When the score is 3 or 4, the clinician has two options: the patient could be kept under observation and repeat the tests or, even more, order additional tests such as an US or a CT scan if they are available in that particular setting. Another option is to rely on the clinical impression of the examiner because, as I already mentioned in my original article, "there is always an intangible ingredient in the diagnosis of acute appendicitis."

The modified Alvarado score (MAS) [2] is a simplification of the Alvarado score by eliminating the neutrophil count because a differential WBC count is not available in certain facilities. The results are similar to the original score but with less capacity to detect the early stages of acute appendicitis.

The Pediatric Appendicitis Score (PAS), developed by Samuel in 2002 [3], is a modification of the Alvarado score in which the rebound sign has been replaced by cough/percussion/hopping tenderness in the right lower quadrant, and the elevation of temperature has been increased to 38°C. In this score the sign of tenderness in the right lower quadrant, the most relevant feature of the score, was given one point only.

The Appendicitis Inflammatory Response (AIR) score [4] is based along the same principles of the Alvarado score assigning patients to low, medium, or high probability of acute appendicitis. It was developed by Andersson and Andersson in 2008 and was constructed from eight independent variables (right lower quadrant pain, rebound tenderness, muscular defense, WBC count, proportion of neutrophils, CRP, body temperature, and vomiting). The AIR score contains rebound tenderness or muscular defense that is divided in three groups—light, medium, and strong—which makes these signs subjective and very difficult to evaluate, and this may deviate the final score one way or another. Besides this, the AIR score omits the symptom of migration of pain which is a very important and specific symptom in the diagnosis of acute appendicitis.

The Raja Isteri Pengiran Anak Saleha Appendicitis (RIPASA) score [5] was developed for the diagnosis of acute appendicitis in Brunei, Darussalam, in 2008. It contains 14 patient characteristics: gender, age, and symptoms, right iliac fossa (RIF) pain, migration to the RIF, anorexia, nausea and vomiting, duration of symptoms, and clinical signs RIF tenderness, guarding, rebound tenderness, Rovsing sign, and fever. It also contains two laboratory tests (WBC and urinalysis) and an additional parameter related to a foreign national card record. Some authors found that the Alvarado score was disappointing in the diagnosis of acute appendicitis in Asian and Mid-Eastern populations, so they decided to have a different score more suitable to them. Chong [6] found that the RIPASA score of >7.5 correctly classified 98% patients confirmed with histological findings of acute appendicitis in comparison with 68.3% patients with an Alvarado score of >7. However, RIPASA and Alvarado scores correctly classified 81.3% and 87.9% patients without acute appendicitis into the true negative groups with scores of >7.5 and <7, respectively. The negative appendectomy rate was 14.66% for the RIPASA score and 13.75% for the Alvarado score.

Khadda et al. [7] found that the RIPASA score has a sensitivity of 97.7% and a specificity of 77.4% and a negative appendectomy rate of 13.7% which is higher than many reports that had used the Alvarado score such as Menon et al. [8], in Pakistan, who reported a negative appendectomy rate of 1.9%. In other study, Pouget-Baudry et al. [9], in France, reported 3 out of 174 patients with a normal appendix on histological examination which equals to 1.72%. The good thing is that Khadda recognized that the Alvarado score is the simplest of all the scores used in current practice. Furthermore, Gaikwad et al. [10], in India, found that the false-positive rate is reduced to zero when ultrasonography is added to the Alvarado score.

Goel et al. [11], in India, evaluated the efficacy of the Alvarado score and the RIPASA score finding that the Alvarado score has a better specificity than the RIPASA score (100 vs. 50%) and also a better negative appendectomy rate (0 vs. 5%). Similar results were reported by Karami et al. [12], in Iran, who found that the Alvarado score was 100% specific as compared with the RIPASA and the AIR scores (91.6% for both).

Malik et al. [13], in Ireland, found that the RIPASA score has a PPV of 84.06% and a NPV of 72.86% with a negative appendectomy rate of 15.94% and an accuracy of 80%. This is the first study evaluating the utility of the RIPASA score predicting acute appendicitis in a Western population. However, Rodrigues and Sindhu [14], in India, found that the Alvarado score had a greater specificity, PPV, and positive likelihood than the RIPASA score. The negative appendectomy in this study was quite high (18.09%) as compared to different negative appendectomy rates reported with the Alvarado score that range between 0 and 10%. Similar results were reported by Rathod et al. [15] with a negative appendectomy rate of 20.69% and a perforated appendicitis of 8.05%. This indicates that the RIPASA score can reduce the number of complicated appendectomies at the expense of a high negative appendectomy rate.

In a recent study in India, Regar et al. [16] found that the Alvarado score is more specific (80%) than the RIPASA score (60%). The PPV of the Alvarado score was 98.46% as compared to 97.83% of the RIPASA score. The negative appendectomy rate for the Alvarado score was lower that the RIPASA score (1.54 vs. 2.17%).

In another recent study, Sinnet et al. [17], in India, found that the RIPASA score has more sensitivity than the Alvarado score (95.5 vs. 65%) but has less specificity (65 vs. 90%). The PPV was 92.89% for the RIPASA score and 96.6% for the Alvarado score which indicates that the negative appendectomy rate is higher for the RIPASA score than the Alvarado score (7.61 vs. 3.33%).

In a study to assess the reliability and practical application of the Alvarado, Eskelinen, Ohmann, and RIPASA scoring systems, Erdem et al. [18], in Turkey, found that the Alvarado score had the best negative appendectomy rate (12%) than the RIPASA score (25%). The negative appendectomy rate for the Ohmann and the Eskelinen scores was 22 and 21%, respectively.

Diaz-Barrientos et al. [19], in Mexico, found that the RIPASA score showed no advantage over the Modified Alvarado score taking into consideration that the ROC curve area was 0.59 for the RIPASA score vs. 0.71 for the modified Alvarado score.

In another study, in Mexico, Reyes-Garcia et al. [20] found 15.7% cases of necrotic appendicitis and 14.3% cases of perforated appendix when using the RIPASA score. The negative appendectomy rate was also high (18.6%).

Golden et al. [21] compared the physician-determined decision with the RIPASA, the Alvarado, and the modified Alvarado score systems in order to measure the physician gestalt in the diagnosis of acute appendicitis. They found that at the higher "rule-in" cutoff threshold, the RIPASA score had a high sensitivity (78%) but a low specificity (36%). Conversely, the modified Alvarado score had a low sensitivity (47%) and a high specificity (81%). The original Alvarado score had test characteristics between these two values. They also calculated the test characteristics for the clinical scoring systems at lower "rule-out" threshold. The NPV for each score varied from 75% for the modified Alvarado score to 89% for the RIPASA score. The NPV for the physician-determined decision was 83%. The area under the curve (AUC) was greatest for the Alvarado score and the physician-determined decision (72% for both), 70% for the MAS score, and 67% for the RIPASA score. These authors concluded that the physician-determined probability estimates were accurate as these scoring systems, which proves that the physician gestalt works well in the diagnosis of acute appendicitis.

All of these findings on the RIPASA score indicate that we need more studies to find out why the differences among the Western and South Asian and Middle Eastern populations. It is possible that these differences have to do with the anatomical position of the appendix and not precisely with the physiopathological process of acute appendicitis or the cultural differences of these populations.

2. Other scores

There are other less-known scores similar to the Alvarado score such as the Adult Appendicitis score of Sammalkorpi et al. [22] that was constructed by logistic regression analysis using multiple imputations for missing values. This score contains four symptoms and clinical signs including the sign of guarding divided into three graduations (mild, moderate, and severe) which is in reality a very subjective sign. It also contains two laboratory tests (WBC and CRP) divided at different levels that are very difficult to memorize. They reported sensitivities and specificities similar to the Alvarado score and areas under the ROC curve of 0.882 for the new score and 0.790 for the Alvarado score. The negative appendectomy rate for this new score is 18.2% which is much higher than the usual reported rates with the Alvarado score.

The Tzanakis scoring system [23] is a very simplified score that contains two clinical signs only: right abdominal tenderness (four points) and rebound tenderness (three points). The only laboratory test is a white blood cell count (WBC) greater than 12.000 cells/mm^3 (two points). The score relies on positive ultrasound scan findings (six points).

Sigdel et al. [24] carried out a prospective study of the Tzanakis score to compare this score with the Alvarado score and reported a sensitivity of 91.4% for the Tzanakis score and 81% for the Alvarado score. The specificity for both scores was the same (66.6%). The ROC curve gave an AUC of 0.867 for the Tzanakis score and 0.81 for the Alvarado score. The negative appendectomy rate was reported as 6% which is certainly low and is due to the addition of the ultrasound studies that are not available in many health facilities. The overall diagnostic accuracy for the Tzanakis score was 91.48% vs. 81.91% for the Alvarado score.

In a study to compare the sensitivity, specificity, and diagnostic accuracy of the Tzanakis score (TS) and the modified Alvarado score (MAS), Sharma et al. [25], in India, found that the sensitivity for the MAS was higher than the TS score (97.7 vs. 82.0%), but the specificity for the TS was higher (36.38 vs. 18%). The PPV for both scores was the same (19%), and the accuracy for the MAS was better than the TS (89 vs. 79%). They concluded that the MAS was better than the TS since in the TS there are chances of observer bias. Besides this, they could not wait till a leukocyte count goes up to 12,000 cells/cm^3 if clinical suspicion is present.

Kumar et al. [26], in India, found that the Tzanakis score is an effective modality in the establishment of accuracy in the diagnosis of acute appendicitis, but the limitation is observer bias which may vary the scoring results.

The Lintula score [27] was developed from 35 symptoms and clinical signs recorded for 131 Finnish children with abdominal pain and was modeled using logistic regression. This complicated score uses gender, intensity of pain, relocation of pain, vomiting, pain in the right lower quadrant, fever, guarding, bowel sounds, and rebound tenderness with different grades. Some of these signs are very difficult to evaluate which may alter the final scoring.

Konan et al. [28], in a study to compare the Alvarado and the Lintula scores in patients older than 65 years of age, found that the Alvarado score was better predictor than the Lintula score. Both scores have a high sensitivity and specificity in the diagnosis of acute appendicitis.

Ojuka and Sangoro [29], in a prospective study, carried out at Kenyatta National Hospital, found that the ROC curves for Lintula and Alvarado scores are almost identical (0.6824 and 0.6966), respectively. However, the sensitivity for the Lintula score is lower than the Alvarado score (60.8 vs. 83.3%), and the overall accuracy for the Lintula score was also lower (69.6 vs. 70.4%).

The Ohmann score [30] was developed in Germany using a computer-aided diagnosis. The variables of the score are tenderness, no micturition difficulties, steady pain, leukocytosis count >10,000 cells/mm^3, age >50 years, relocation of pain to the right lower quadrant, and rigidity. In spite of this computerized system, there was no improvement in the number of perforations or complications.

In an analysis of scores in the diagnosis of acute appendicitis in women, Horzić et al. [31] compared the modified Alvarado score, Ohmann score, and Eskelinen score finding that all patients with the modified Alvarado score of 7 or more had acute appendicitis (100% specificity) which can be used to determine the need for immediate appendectomy.

Recently, Wilasrusmee et al. [32] developed a new appendicitis score for patients with suspected appendicitis and compared it with the Alvarado score. This score, also known as RAMA-AS, includes seven variables (migration of pain, progression of pain, pain aggravation by cough or movement, temperature of 37.8°C or more, and rebound tenderness). Also, it includes two laboratory tests (WBC >10,000 cells/mm^3 and neutrophils <75%). In the evaluation of the variables of the score, there are serious questions. For example, they gave great importance to rebound tenderness (the only sign of the score) which contradicts the literature that always mentions direct tenderness in the right lower quadrant as the main variable. Besides this, their own statistic shows that rebound tenderness is present in 23.9%, whereas tenderness in the right lower quadrant is present in 88.4% of their cases. Another significant discrepancy is that they gave more importance to pain aggravation than anorexia (56.3 vs. 76.1%). Another objectionable symptom is progression of pain since this is a very subjective symptom that is difficult to evaluate. The C-statistics reported by Wilasrusmee et al. are better than the Alvarado score, but the RAMA-AS score did not perform well in the external data when compared to the derived data. Using the score in practice is not as easy as claimed by this group since it requires the use of the Fagan nomogram. In addition, the calculation of the score is difficult to obtain because the evaluation of the parameters is given in fractional numbers. For all of these reasons, the new score will need external evaluations to establish its usefulness in the real practice.

Khanafer et al. [33] made some modifications to the Alvarado score (AS) and the Pediatric Appendicitis score (PAS) to screen children at low risk for appendicitis who could be carefully observed at home without the need for laboratory investigation. In this study, a total of 180 children were enrolled with an average age of 11.2 years of which 56.7% were female. According to their findings, children with a score of >7 for the modified PAS and AS may be safely sent home with close follow-up, while those above this cut-off would benefit from a referral for further evaluation in the ED. They found similar sensitivities for all the scores but reduced specificities and predictive values for the modified PAS and AS scores. As expected, the ROC curves showed a reduced AUC using the modified scores. The negative appendectomy rate was 5.2% only.

3. Conclusion

A good diagnostic score for acute appendicitis should be simple, easy to memorize, repeatable, economical, and easy to apply in an emergency setting. It should contain elements with a good statistical significance. Also, a good diagnostic score for acute appendicitis could be useful for statistical purposes by providing a more precise indexing of the disease. For example, it could be used, as a clinical indicator, in the International Classification of Diseases at a fifth digit level.

Author details

Alfredo Alvarado[1,2,3,4,5*]

*Address all correspondence to: alfredoalvara@hotmail.com

1 Alma Mater Universidad Nacional de Colombia, Bogotá, Colombia

2 Certified by the American Board of Surgeons and the American Board of Emergency Medicine, Miami, FL, USA

3 International College of Surgeons, Chicago, IL, USA

4 Society of Laparoscopic Surgeons, Chicago, USA

5 American College of Emergency Physicians, Irving TX, USA

References

[1] Alvarado A. A practical score for the early diagnostic of acute appendicitis. Annals of Emergency Medicine. 1986;**15**(5):557-564

[2] Kalan M, Talbot D, Cunliffe WJ, Rich AJ. Evaluation of the modified Alvarado score in the diagnosis of acute appendicitis: A prospective study. Annals of the Royal College of Surgeons of England. 1994;**76**:418-419

[3] Samuel M. Pediatric appendicitis score. Journal of Pediatric Surgery. 2002;**37**:877-881

[4] Andersson M, Andersson R. The appendicitis inflammatory response score: A tool for the diagnosis of acute appendicitis that outperforms the Alvarado score. World Journal of Surgery. 2008;**32**:1843-1849

[5] Chong CF, Adi MI, Thien A, et al. Development of the RIPASA score: A new appendicitis scoring system for the diagnosis of acute appendicitis. Singapore Medical Journal. 2018;**51**:220-225

[6] Chong CF, Thien A, Mackie AJA, et al. Comparison of RIPASA and Alvarado scores for the diagnosis of acute appendicitis. Singapore Medical Journal. 2011;**52**(5):340-345

[7] Khadda S, Yadav AK, Anwar A, et al. Clinical study to evaluate the RIPASA scoring system in the diagnosis of acute appendicitis. American Journal of Advanced Medical and Surgical Research. 2015;**1**(29):67-73

[8] Menon AA, Vohra LM, Khalik T, Lehri AA. Diagnostic accuracy of Alvarado score in the diagnosis of acute appendicitis. Pakistan Journal of Medical Sciences. Jan 2009;**25**(1): 118-121

[9] Pouget-Baudry Y, Mucci S, Eyssartier E. Le score clinicobiologique d'Alvarado dans la prise en charge d'une douleur de fosse iliaque droite chez l'adulte. Journal de Chirurgie Viscerale. Apr 2010;**147**(2):128-132

[10] Gaikwad V, Murchite S, Chandra S, Modi P. To evaluate the efficacy of Alvarado score and ultrasonography in acute appendicitis. Journal of Dental and Medical Sciences. Sep 2016;**15**(9):14-18

[11] Goel P, Mishra K, Sharma, et al. The study to evaluate the efficacy of Alvarado score and RIPASA score in diagnosis of acute appendicitis and correlation with intraoperative and pathological findings. Annals of Medical and Dental Research. Oct 2017;**3**(6):33-39

[12] Karami MY, Niakan H, Zabedagheri N, et al. Which one is better? Comparison of acute inflammatory response, Raja Isteri Pengiran Anak Saleha appendicitis and alvarado scoring systems. Annals of Coloproctology. Dec 2017;**33**(6):227-231

[13] Malik MU, Connelly TM, Awan F, et al. The RIPASA score is sensitive and specific for the diagnosis of acute appendicitis in a western population. International Journal of Colorectal Disease. Apr 2017;**32**(4):491-494

[14] Rodrigues W, Sindhu S. Diagnostic importance of Alvarado score in acute appendicitis. International Journal of Scientific Study. Feb 2017;**4**(11):57-60

[15] Rathod S, Ali I, Bawa A, et al. Evaluation of Raja Isteri Pengiran Anak Saleha appendicitis scoring system. Medical Journal of D.Y. Patil University. 2015;**8**:744-749

[16] Regar MK, Choudhary GS, Nogia C, et al. Comparison of Alvarado and RIPASA scoring systems in diagnosis of acute appendicitis and correlation with intraoperative and histopathological findings. International Journal of Surgery. May 2017;**4**(5):1755-1761

[17] Sinnet P, Chellappa KS, et al. Comparative study on the diagnostic accuracy of the RIPASA score over Alvarado score in the diagnosis of acute appendicitis. Journal of Evidence Based Medicine Healthcare. 2016;**3**(80):4318-4321

[18] Erdem F, Cetincünar S, Dag K, et al. Alvarado, Esleinem, Ohmann and Raja Isteri Pengiran Anak Saleha appendicitis scores for diasgnosis of acute appendicitis. World Journal of Gastroenterology. Dec 2013;**1947**(47):9057-9062

[19] Diaz-Barrientos CZ, Aquino-Gonzalez A, Heredia-Montaño M, et al. Escala RIPASA para el diagnóstico de apendicitis aguda: Comparación con la escala de Alvarado. Revista de Gastroenterología de México. Feb 2018. Article in press (5 pages)

[20] Reyes-Garcia N, Zaldivar-Ramirez FR, Cruz-Martinez R, et al. Precisión diagnóstica de la escala de RIPASA para el diagnóstico de apendicitis aguda: análisis comparativo con la escala de Alvarado modificada. Cirujano General. Apr-Jun 2012;**34**(2):101-106

[21] Golden SK, Harringa JB, Pickhard PJ, et al. Prospective evaluation of the ability of clinical scoring systems and physician-determined likelihood of appendicitis to obviate the need for CT. Emergency Medicine Journal. 2016;**0**:1-7

[22] Sammalkorpi MP, Leppaniemi P. A new adult appendicitis score improves diagnostic accuracy of acute appendicitis: A prospective study. BMC Gastroenterology. 2014;**14**:114

[23] Tzanakis NE, Stamatis P, Danulidis K, et al. New approach to accurate diagnosis of acute appendicitis. World Journal of Surgery. 2005;**29**(9):1151-1155

[24] Sigdel GS, Lakhey PJ, Mishra PR. Tzanakis score vs Alvarado score in acute appendicitis. Journal of the Nepal Medical Association. Apr-Jun 2010;**49**(178):96-99

[25] Sharma A, Gharde P, Gharbe PM, et al. European Journal of Biomedical and Pharmaceutical Sciences. 2017;**4**(4):588-559

[26] Kumar SLA, Nagaraja AL, Srinivasaiah M. Evaluation of Tzanakis scoring system in acute appendicitis. International Journal of Surgery. Oct 2017;**4**(10):3338-3343

[27] Lintula H, Kokki H, Ketunnen R, Eskelinen M. Appendicitis score for children with suspected appendicitis. A randomized clinical trial. Langenbeck's Archives of Surgery. Nov 2009;**294**(6):999-1004

[28] Konan A, Hayran M, Kilic YA. Scoring systems in the diagnosis of acute appendicitis in the elderly. Ulusal Travma ve Acil Cerrahi Dergisi. Oct 2011;**17**(5):396-400

[29] Ojuka D, Sangoro M. Alvarado vs Lintula scoring system in acute appendicitis. The Annals of African Surgery. Jan 2017;**14**(1):21-25

[30] Ohmann C, Franke C, Yang Q. Clinical benefit of a diagnostic score for appendicitis: Results of a prospective interventional study. Archives of Surgery. 1999;**134**(9):993-996

[31] Horzic M, Salamon A, Kopljar M, et al. Analysis of scores in diagnosis of acute appendicitis in women. Collegium Antropologicum. 2005;**29**(1):133-138

[32] Wilasrusmee C, Sirimbumrungwong P, et al. Developing and validating of Ramathibodi appendicitis score (RAMA-AS) for diagnosis of appendicitis in suspected appendicitis patients. World Journal of Emergency Surgery. 2017;**12**:49

[33] Khanafer et al. Test characteristics of common appendicitis scores with and without laboratory investigations: A prospective observational study. BMC Pediatrics. Aug 30, 2016; **16**(1):147

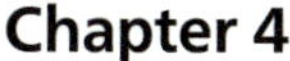

Chapter 4

Imaging in Suspected Appendicitis

Jaime A. Fandiño Romero and
Fernando Meléndez Negrette

Additional information is available at the end of the chapter

http://dx.doi.org/10.5772/intechopen.75035

Abstract

Appendicitis is the most suspected diagnosis in patients who consult for abdominal pain, and appendicitis is the most common cause which requires urgent abdominal surgery or intervention. Classically, the diagnosis has been made with the patient's medical history, physical examination, and laboratory findings; however, its preoperative diagnosis is increasingly reliant on imaging. The negative appendectomy rates decreased after the introduction of the use of imaging modalities. The diagnosis of appendicitis should be made early to avoid complications such as perforation. The objective of this chapter is to describe briefly the most important findings in each available image modality and the impact they have on the management and list the potential mimics of appendicitis.

Keywords: appendicitis, compression ultrasound, multidetector computed tomography, magnetic resonance imaging, abdominal imaging

1. Introduction

Appendicitis in a common surgical problem is the most frequent cause of acute abdominal pain [1].

Using the clinical scoring system Alvarado with a low score of 1–4 only, some patients should be considered for imaging. Those with Alvarado score of 5–7 should have imaging performed [2].

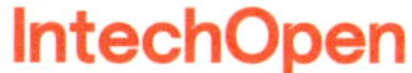

2. Diagnostic imaging

In all patients who have clinical suspicion of appendicitis, we have various modalities of images to either confirm the diagnosis or rule out other causes of abdominal pain and reduce the rate of negative appendectomies such as ultrasound (US), computed tomography (CT), magnetic resonance, and conventional radiography in some cases.

In this chapter we will review the most common findings in each modality of diagnostic imaging.

It is important to know the normal location of the appendix to know where we can find it at the diagnostic images; the location of the base is relatively constant, while the location of the tip is more variable due to its variable length.

The tip of the appendix will be located behind the cecum (ascending retrocecal) 65%, inferior to the cecum (subcecal) 31%, behind the cecum (transverse retrocecal) 2%, anterior to the ileum (ascending paracecal preileal) 1%, and posterior to the ileum (ascending paracecal retroileal) 0.5% [3].

2.1. Conventional radiography

They are not of routine use for the diagnosis of acute appendicitis due to their low specificity. The main finding in this imaging method is the presence of appendicolith, which is visible in less than 5% of patients with acute appendicitis, and its presence does not always indicate acute appendicitis and is not indicative of prophylactic appendectomy in children and adults.

Other nonspecific findings are abnormal gas pattern in the right iliac fossa, gas pattern in the right lower quadrant (ileocecal part or ascending colon topography) of the Klemm's sign [4], the presence of a sentinel loop, and loss of the right psoas margin. The use of barium would show indirect signs such as lack of filling of the appendiceal lumen or extrinsic impression of the cecum by an appendiceal abscess [5–8].

2.2. Ultrasound (US)

Ultrasound has had many advances in the last 30 years, and although it is a dependent operator, it is quite useful in the pediatric population and pregnant women for not using ionizing radiation; it has a very low cost and is very accessible.

The ultrasound has a sensitivity of 78 and 83% and a specificity of 83 and 93% [9], which is similar to those reported for physical examination or validated clinical scores such as the Alvarado score, but this one is variable and depends on age; an Alvarado score cut point of 5 was good at "ruling out" admission for appendicitis with a sensitivity of 99% overall (96 men, 99 women, and 99% children). At a cut point of 7 (historically recommended for "ruling in" appendicitis and progression to surgery), the score performed poorly with specificity overall of 81% (men 57, women 73, and children 76%). The Alvarado score was well calibrated in men; however, it tended to overpredict appendicitis in women and children subgroups. The standard Alvarado scoring is useful in areas with limited resources and no imaging diagnostic tools [10].

In the graded compression technique described by Puylaert in 1986 with a linear high-frequency transducer, pressure is applied in order to displace gas-filled loops of bowel [11]. Another technique can be used, like left lateral decubitus position for retrocecal position. About 23% of normal appendices are larger than 6 mm according to one ultrasound-based study; for this reason some institutions use a threshold of 7 mm [12].

The ultrasound findings are aperistaltic, noncompressible, dilated appendix (>6–7 mm outer diameter), one or more appendicoliths with echogenic shadowing foci, target appearance in axial section, distinct appendiceal wall layers (**Figure 1**), and occasionally extra-appendiceal changes like echogenic prominent pericecal and periappendiceal fat, hyperechoic structure surrounding a noncompressible appendix (**Figure 2**), and periappendiceal reactive nodal enlargement or fluid collection [13].

Color Doppler ultrasound shows increased vascularity (**Figure 3**) or decreased if ischemia is present.

In the description of the severity of inflammation real time ultrasound elastography can be useful [14].

The limitations and disadvantages of the ultrasound are well known like it is operator dependent and requires years of training. The appendix is not always visualizable especially in retrocecal position and the presence of bowel gas. Another limitation is the reduced penetration of ultrasound in obese patients.

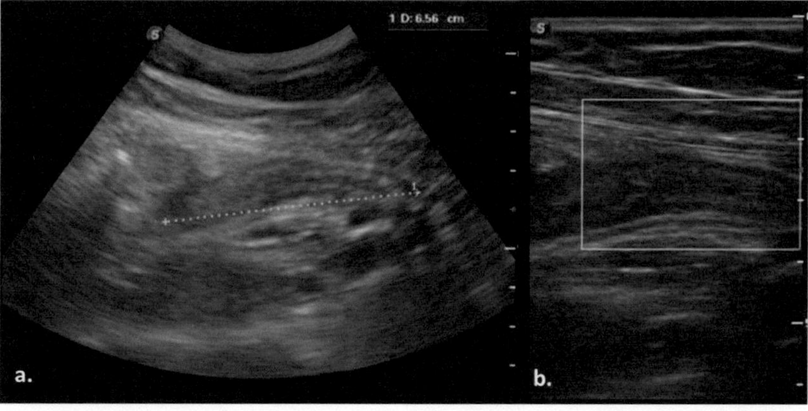

Figure 1. Graded compression sonography images in longitudinal sections (a) of an enlarged, noncompressible appendix compatible with no complicated appendicitis. Color Doppler flow image (b) demonstrated increased blood flow in the wall of the inflamed appendix due to hyperemia.

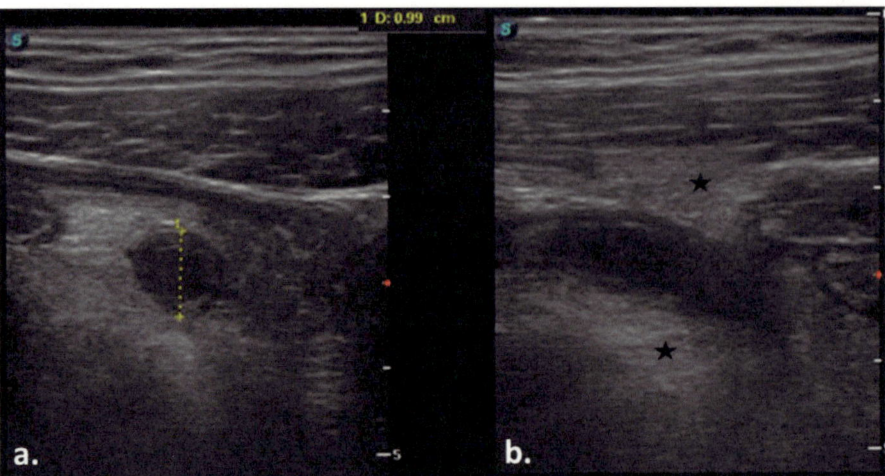

Figure 2. (a) Target appearance (axial section) of periappendiceal hyperechoic structure: Amorphous hyperechoic structure (usually >10 mm) seen surrounding a noncompressible appendix with a diameter of >6 mm. (b) Thickened appendix in longitudinal image and echogenic prominent periappendiceal fat (blacks stars).

2.3. Multidetector CT

For evaluating patients with signs and symptoms of acute appendicitis, controversy about which CT protocol is better exists, and the use of intravenous (IV), oral, and rectal contrast agents is debated. The options include the use of intravenous contrast material alone, oral contrast material alone, rectal contrast material alone, or no contrast material at all [15].

The use of oral contrast material has advantages like allowing a decreased number of false negatives, and appendiceal filling is suggestive of non-obstructed appendix. The disadvantages are increase in the scanning time and delay patient care, the oral contrast can mask appendicoliths, discomfort for the patient, and higher cost of the imaging examination.

At our hospital, patients with suspected appendicitis undergo CT without contrast material. What is important is that the chosen protocol should be appropriate for each particular patient.

Minimize the patient's exposure to radiation as much as possible; applying ALARA (as low as reasonably achievable) principle is always recommendable [16].

The sensitivity and specificity of CT are high (94–98%) and specific (up to 97%), respectively, for the diagnosis of acute appendicitis and can help for differential diagnosis [17].

CT diagnosis of appendicitis can include some of these findings like dilated appendix (>6 mm), thickening and enhancing of the wall, and thickening of the cecal apex (**Figure 4**) and extra-appendiceal findings like extraluminal fluid, abscess formation, appendicolith (**Figure 5**), and periappendiceal inflammation, including stranding of the adjacent fat (**Figure 6**) and thickening of the lateroconal fascia or mesoappendix or reactive nodal enlargement [18].

For the differentiation of complicated from uncomplicated, the CT plays an important role.

http://dx.doi.org/10.5772/intechopen.75035

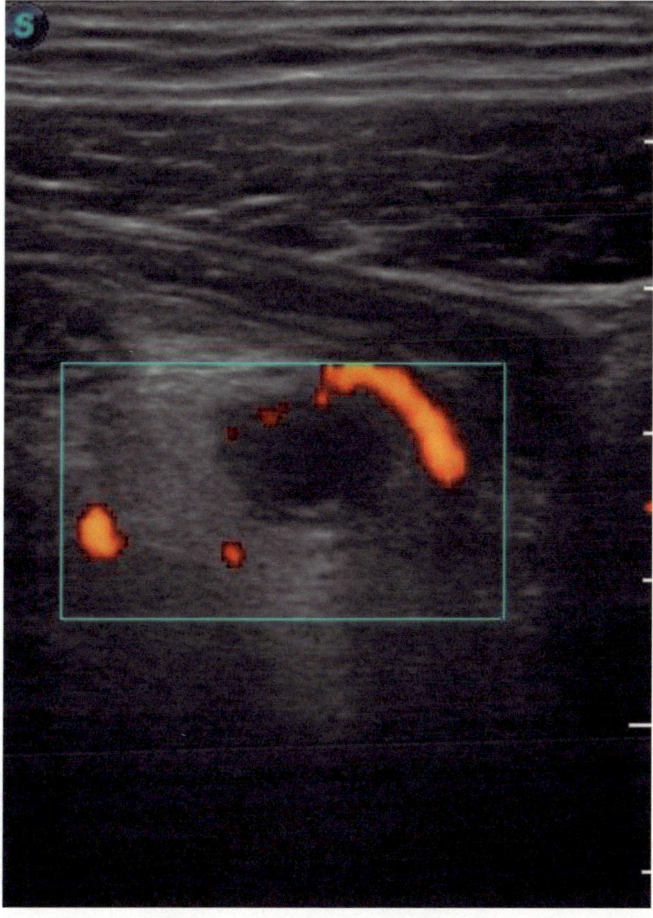

Figure 3. Axial US image with power Doppler shows increased vascularity.

Although it may be difficult to differentiate a simple appendicitis from a perforated appendicitis, there are some classics of CT findings of perforated appendicitis like extraluminar air, the presence of one or more extraluminar appendicolith, abscess, phlegmon, and defect in mural enhancement (highest sensitivity at 64%); these five findings collectively have a 95% of sensitivity and specificity for a diagnosis of perforated appendicitis [19].

2.4. Magnetic resonance imaging

Magnetic resonance imaging (MRI) is not commonly used to diagnose appendicitis but lacks of effects of ionizing radiation, which makes it ideal for pregnant patients and children with symptoms of appendicitis and equivocal US findings.

In pregnant patients, the clinical diagnosis of appendicitis can be difficult, the location of pain may be atypical, and the classics symptoms are nonspecific. A negative appendectomy is associated with a higher risk of fetal loss and premature delivery.

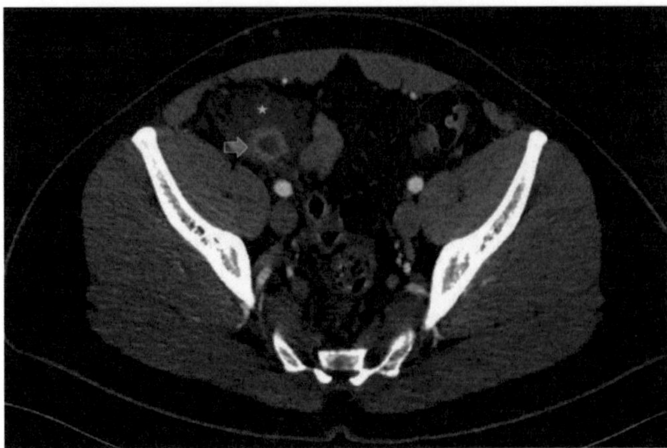

Figure 4. Axial Multidetector CT (MDCT) image with intravenous contrast in a man with suspected appendicitis. The appendix (white arrowheads) is fluid filled, showing an increased caliber (>6 mm) (target sign), extra-appendiceal findings of periappendiceal inflammation, and stranding of the adjacent fat (white star).

The appendix can be difficult to visualize with ultrasound in a pregnant patient, MRI has excellent anatomic resolution, and it is safe in these patients.

MRI is most expensive, takes longer time to be performed, and also can be degraded by motion artifacts.

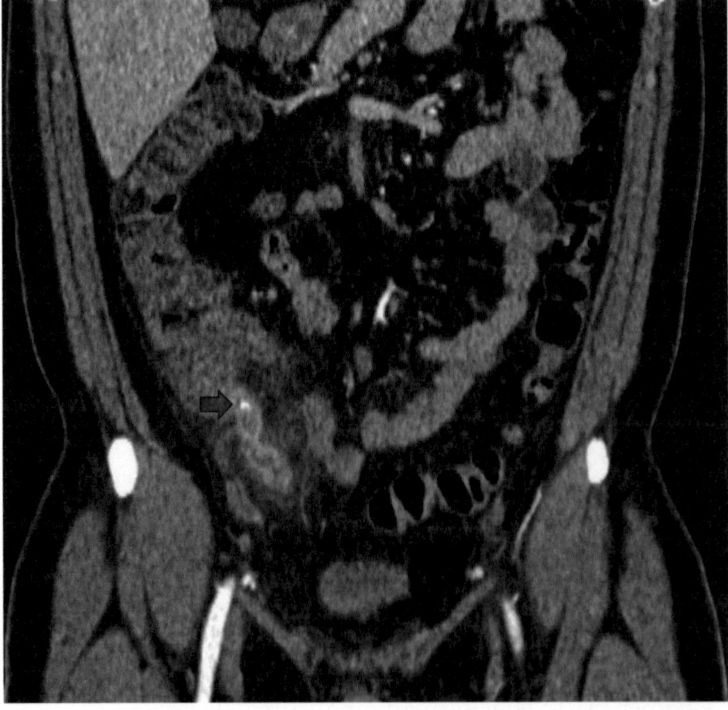

Figure 5. Coronal CT with intravenous contrast image showing the presence of an appendicolith on the same patient (white arrow).

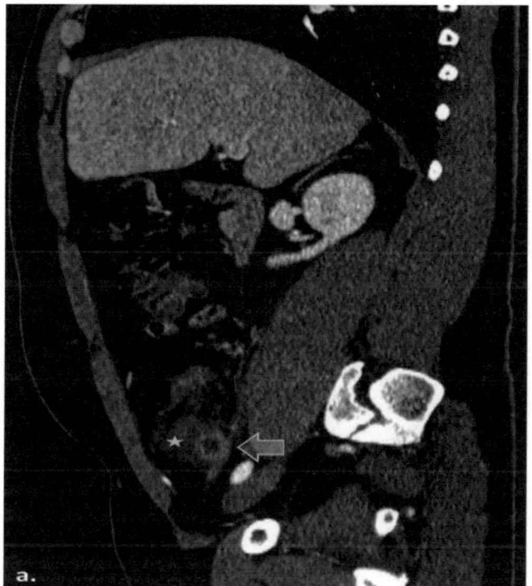

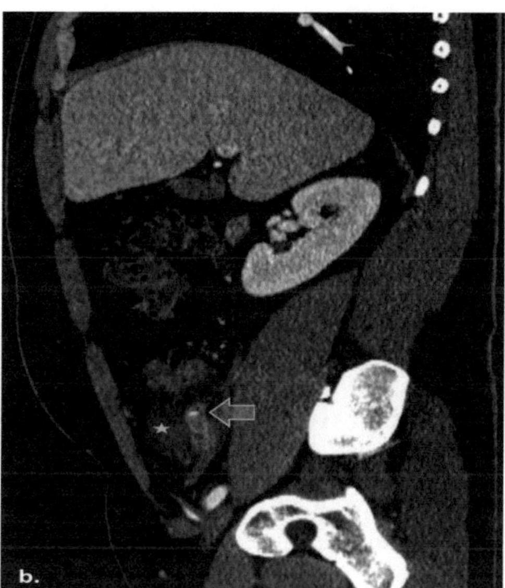

Figure 6. Sagittal CT image: (a) the appendix (white arrowheads) shows target sign, periappendiceal inflammation, and stranding of the adjacent fat (white star). (b) Appendicolith.

MRI is considered to provide positive results for acute appendicitis when the appendix is enlarged (>7 mm), the appendiceal wall is thicker than 2 mm, or there are signs of inflammatory changes (**Figure 7**).

It is important to remind that although MRI is safe during pregnancy and no fetal effects have been documented, no IV contrast should be used during pregnancy because gadolinium is a category C drug (potentially teratogenic) [20].

MRI is a promising modality in the evaluation of suspected acute appendicitis despite the fact that its reliability in differentiating perforated from simple appendicitis has considered in some

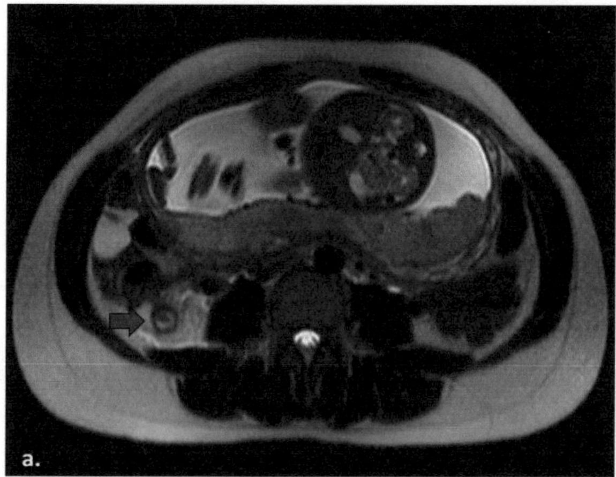

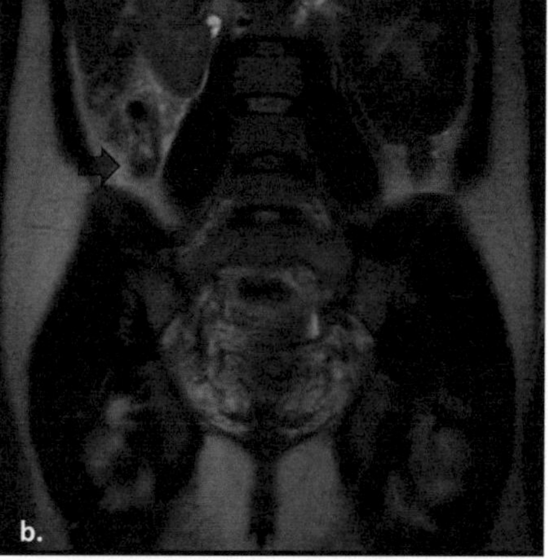

Figure 7. (a) Axial and (b) coronal MR scan with T2-weighted coronal image of the abdomen in a gravid woman. Arrow highlights the thickened appendix.

cases unsatisfactory and MRI findings predictive of appendiceal perforation have not been specifically evaluated clearly; some authors recently have established that contrast-enhanced MRI can differentiate perforated from non-perforated appendicitis in pediatric population based on the appendiceal diameter and another MRI finding like appendiceal restricted diffusion, wall defect, appendicolith, periappendiceal free fluid, remote free fluid, restricted diffusion within free fluid, abscess, peritoneal enhancement, ileocecal wall thickening, and ileus. Abscess, wall defect, and restricted diffusion within free fluid had the greatest specificity for perforation but low sensitivity, and a threshold of any four findings mentioned had the best ability to accurately discriminate between perforated and non-perforated cases, with a sensitivity of 82% and specificity of 85% [21].

3. Complicated appendicitis

One of the main objectives of the diagnostic images is to contribute to the early diagnosis to avoid possible complications, and the differentiation of complicated from uncomplicated is important to define the definitive treatment. The possible complications include perforation which we have already mentioned and the role of computated tomography, ultrasound, to

US	CT
ACUTE APPENDICITIS	
Enlarged appendix(greater than 6 mm)	Enlarged appendix
Wall thickening	Wall thickening
Appendicolith	Appendicolith
Target sign	Target sign
Periappendiceal lymphadenopathy	Periappendiceal lymphadenopathy
Blind ending aperistaltic tubular structure	Periappendiceal fat strading
	Wall enhancement
	Focal apical thickening
PERFORATED APPENDICITIS	
Appendiceal wall defect	Appendiceal wall defect
Abscess	Abscess
Extraluminal appendicolith	Extraluminal appendicolith
Periappendiceal fluid collection	Periappendiceal fluid collection
	Extraliminar air
	Phlegmon

Table 1. CT and ultrasound findings of simple and perforated appendicitis.

differentiate between simple and perforated appendicitis are listed in **Table 1**; another complication can include abscess, peritonitis, pylephlebitis and pylethrombosis, genitourinary involvement(hydronephrosis), and gangrenous appendicitis(pneumatosis, shaggy appendiceal wall, and patchy areas of mural nonperfusion) [22]. Other complications can be bowel obstruction, chronic and recurrent appendicitis, or rare complication like fistulation [23].

4. Secondary or reactive appendicitis

There are some inflammatory conditions that can lead to the development of appendicitis, and although they are not frequent, it is important to mention them; each of these entities has specific findings in the diagnostic images affecting the appendix, and computed tomography plays a fundamental role by differentiating each of them.

The causes of secondary appendicitis can be Crohn's disease, diverticulitis, colitis, terminal ileitis, and gynecologic causes like tubo-ovarian abscess or pyosalpinx.

For all these entities, the clinical context associated with the appendicular involvement evidenced by images is of vital importance for the diagnosis.

5. Differential diagnosis

Differential diagnosis can include mesenteric adenitis (clinically the most common differential and most frequent in children and adolescents), and features on CT and ultrasound include enlarged lymph nodes (three or more), normal appendix if can be identified, and ileal or ileocecal wall thickening [24, 25].

Other differentials can be enlarged normal appendix (50 of asymptomatic patients can have an appendix diameter greater than 6 mm on CT), Crohn's disease, appendiceal mucocele, pelvic inflammatory disease (PID), acute epiploic appendagitis, omental infarction, Meckel's diverticulitis right-sided diverticulitis, and appendiceal neoplasms (carcinoid, metastases, and others) [26].

Except for mesenteric adenitis in children, tomography is the modality of choice that allows us to perform an adequate differential diagnosis.

6. Conclusion

Appendicitis is still one of the most common diagnoses in emergency rooms, the Alvarado score has a good diagnostic utility at specific cutoff points, and after performing a clinical diagnosis, the imaging in these patients with suspected appendicitis has become almost mandatory; the choice of one modality of image or another depends on the profile and context of each patient, ultrasound as being very important in the pediatric population and pregnant women. MRI is important if the ultrasound is nondiagnostic. CT is the modality of choice for most adults and can perform an adequate differential diagnosis.

Acknowledgments

Thanks, all people for being there for us always. To my son for being infinite inspiration.

Conflict of interest

We have no conflict of interest to declare.

Author details

Jaime A. Fandiño Romero* and Fernando Meléndez Negrette

*Address all correspondence to: jaimeandresfr@hotmail.com

Radiology Department, Hospital of the Universidad Del Norte, Barranquilla, Colombia

References

[1] Birnbaum BA, Wilson SR. Appendicitis at the millennium. Radiology. 2000;**215**(2):337-348

[2] Alvarado A. A practical score for the early diagnosis of acute appendicitis. Annals of Emergency Medicine. 1986 May;**15**(5):557-564

[3] Fritsch H, Kühnel W. Color Atlas of Human Anatomy, Internal Organs. New York, NY, USA: Thieme Medical Publishers; 2008 ISBN:3135334058

[4] White FA. Physical Signs in Medicine and Surgery: An Atlas of Rare, Lost and Forgotten. Xlibris: United States; 2009

[5] Baker SR. Acute appendicitis: Plain radiographic considerations. Emergency Radiology. 1996;**3**:63-69

[6] Parks NA, Schroeppel TJ. Update on imaging for acute appendicitis. The Surgical Clinics of North America. 2011;**91**:14154

[7] Schwartz D. Imaging of suspected appendicitis: Appropriateness of various imaging modalities. Pediatric Annals. 2008;**37**:433-438

[8] Ahn SH, Mayo-Smith WW, Murphy BL, et al. Acute nontraumatic abdominal pain in adult patients: Abdominal radiography compared with CT evaluation. Radiology. 2002; **225**:159-164

[9] Van Randen A, Bipat S, Zwinderman AH, et al. Acute appendicitis: Meta-analysis of diagnostic performance of CT and graded compression US related to prevalence of disease. Radiology. 2008;**249**:97-106

[10] Ohle R, O'reilly F, O'brien KK, Fahey T, Dimitrov BD. The Alvarado score for predicting acute appendicitis: A systematic review. BMC Medicine. 2011;**9**:139

[11] Puylaert JB. Acute appendicitis: US evaluation using graded compression. Radiology. 1986;**158**:355-360

[12] Rettenbacher T, Hollerweger A, Macheiner P, et al. Outer diameter of the vermiform appendix as a sign of acute appendicitis: Evaluation at US. Radiology. 2001;**218**:757-762

[13] Noguchi T, Yoshimitsu K, Yoshida M. Periappendiceal hyperechoic structure on sonography: A sign of severe appendicitis. Journal of Ultrasound in Medicine: Official Journal of the American Institute of Ultrasound in Medicine. 2005 Mar;**24**(3):323-327. Quiz 328-330

[14] Kapoor A, Kapoor A, Mahajan G. Real-time elastography in acute appendicitis. Journal of Ultrasound in Medicine. 2010;**29**(6):871-877

[15] Anderson SW, Soto JA, Lucey BC, Ozonoff A, Jordan JD, Ratevosian J, Ulrich AS, Rathlev NK, Mitchell PM, Rebholz C, Feldman JA, Rhea JT. Abdominal 64-MDCT for suspected appendicitis: The use of oral and IV contrast material versus IV contrast material only. AJR. American Journal of Roentgenology. 2009 Nov;**193**(5):1282-1288

[16] Krishnamoorthi R, Ramarajan N, Wang NE, et al. Effectiveness of a staged US and CT protocol for the diagnosis of pediatric appendicitis: Reducing radiation exposure in the age of ALARA. Radiology. 2011;**259**:231-239

[17] Fefferman NR, Roche KJ, Pinkney LP, et al. Suspected appendicitis in children: Focused CT technique for evaluation. Radiology. 2001;**220**:691-695

[18] Pereira JM, Sirlin CB, Pinto PS, et al. Disproportionate fat stranding: A helpful CT sign in patients with acute abdominal pain. Radiographics. 2004;**24**(3):703-715

[19] Horrow MM, White DS, Horrow JC. Differentiation of perforated from nonperforated appendicitis at CT. Radiology. 2003;**227**(1):46-51

[20] Singh A, Danrad R, Hahn PF, et al. MR imaging of the acute abdomen and pelvis: Acute appendicitis and beyond. Radiographics. 2007;**27**:1419-1431

[21] Rosenbaum DG, Askin G, Beneck DM, et al. Differentiating perforated from nonperforated appendicitis on contrast-enhanced magnetic resonance imaging. Pediatric Radiology. 2017;**47**:1483

[22] Pinto Leite N, Pereira JM, Cunha R, Pinto P, Sirlin C. CT evaluation of appendicitis and its complications: Imaging techniques and key diagnostic findings. AJR. American Journal of Roentgenology. 2005;**185**(2):406-417

[23] Singal R, Gupta S, Mittal A, et al. Appendico-cutaneous fistula presenting as a large wound: A rare phenomenon—Brief review. Acta Medica Indonesiana. 2012;**44**(1):53-56

[24] Macari M, Hines J, Balthazar E, et al. Mesenteric adenitis: CT diagnosis of primary versus secondary causes, incidence, and clinical significance in pediatric and adult patients. AJR. American Journal of Roentgenology. 2002;**178**(4):853-858

[25] Lucey BC, Stuhlfaut JW, Soto JA. Mesenteric lymph nodes: Detection and significance on MDCT. AJR. American Journal of Roentgenology. 2005;**184**(1):41-44

[26] Purysko AS, Remer EM, Filho HM, et al. Beyond appendicitis: Common and uncommon gastrointestinal causes of right lower quadrant abdominal pain at multidetector CT. Radiographics. 2011;**31**:927-947

Chapter 5

Delayed Appendectomy is Safe in Patients with Acute Nonperforated Appendicitis

Sung Il Choi

Additional information is available at the end of the chapter

http://dx.doi.org/10.5772/intechopen.76077

Abstract

Objective: The present study examined whether acute nonperforated appendicitis is a surgical emergency requiring immediate intervention or a disease that can be treated with a semielective operation.

Summary of background data: Immediate appendectomy has been the gold standard in the treatment of acute appendicitis because of the risk of pathological progression. However, this time-honored practice has been recently challenged by studies suggesting that appendectomies can be elective in some cases and still result in positive outcomes.

Methods: This was a retrospective study using the charts of patients who underwent an appendectomy for acute appendicitis between January 2007 and February 2012. Patients were divided into two groups for comparison: an immediate group (those who were moved to an operating room within 12 hours after hospital arrival) and a delayed group (those who were moved to an operating room within 12 to 24 hours after hospital arrival). The end points were conversion rate, operative time, perforation rate, complication rate, readmission rate, length of hospital stay, and medical costs.

Results: of 1805 patients, 1342 (74.3%) underwent immediate operation within 12 hours after hospital arrival, whereas 463 (25.7%) underwent delayed operation within 12–24 hours. There were no significant differences in open conversion, operative time, perforation, postoperative complications, and readmission between the two groups. Length of hospital stay was significantly greater (3.7 ± 1.7 days) and medical costs were also greater (2346.3 ± 735.3 US dollar) in the delayed group than in the immediate group (3.1 ± 1.9 days, $p = 0.000$ and 2257.8 ± 723.8 US dollar, $p = 0.026$).

Conclusions: delayed appendectomy is safe for patients with acute nonperforated appendicitis.

Keywords: appendicitis, appendectomy, delay, complications, treatment outcome, safety

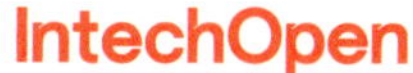

1. Introduction

Acute appendicitis is one of the most common acute diseases requiring an emergency operation. Immediate appendectomy is considered the gold-standard treatment for acute appendicitis. It is widely believed that delays in diagnosis and treatment significantly contribute to increased incidences of perforated appendicitis, which result in increased patient morbidity [1]. Nevertheless, in some cases, the appropriate operation has been delayed because of reasons such as lack of fasting time for general anesthesia, unavailability of operating rooms, and overscheduling of operating teams. Recently, some studies have challenged the impact of these delays and standard of care with appendectomy by suggesting that acute appendicitis can either be treated medically [2, 3] or operated on electively without increasing morbidity [4–7]. Given these considerations, we used electronic medical records to review 1805 cases of appendectomy for acute appendicitis between January 2007 and February 2012 to verify whether acute nonperforated appendicitis necessitates immediate intervention or can be treated with a semielective operation.

2. Methods

2.1. Patients

A retrospective review of the charts of all patients who underwent an appendectomy for acute appendicitis at Kyung Hee University Hospital at Gangdong from January 2007 to February 2012 was performed. Diagnosis of acute non-perforated appendicitis was based on a doctor's decision after considering clinical manifestation, physical examination, laboratory findings, and radiologic modalities. Patients who were preoperatively diagnosed with perforated appendicitis, underwent interval appendectomy or negative appendectomy, or underwent an operation after consulting with other departments were excluded from analysis. Antibiotics such as cephalosporin were administered as soon as possible after diagnosis and were continued until patient discharge. Nowadays, we just give one injection of antibiotics just before surgery. In the case of severe wound complications, we have used antibiotics even if it did not follow guidelines. The data for the following parameters were gathered from electronic medical records: demographic characteristics (age, sex), body mass index (BMI), American Society of Anesthesiologists (ASA) score, white blood cell (WBC) count at admission, body temperature at admission, time from onset of symptoms to hospital arrival (patient interval), time from hospital arrival to the operating room (hospital interval), radiologic findings according to diagnostic modalities, methods of surgery, operative time, and final pathology. The patients were divided into two comparison groups: immediate group (those with a hospital interval ≤12 hours) and delayed group (those with a hospital interval from 12 to 24 hours). The end points chosen for comparison were safety-related outcomes: laparoscopic to open conversion rate, operative time, perforation rate, complication rate, and readmission rate; economy-related outcomes: length of hospital stay and medical cost; and accuracy of diagnostic modalities for distinguishing the difference between nonperforated and perforated appendicitis.

2.2. Statistical analysis

Demographic and clinical characteristics were summarized as means (for continuous variables) or proportions (for categorical variables) and compared using *t* tests or χ^2 tests, respectively. A p value of less than 0.05 was considered statistically significant. All statistical analyses were performed using Statistical Package for Social Sciences (SPSS) software version 18.03 (SPSS Inc., Chicago, IL).

3. Results

3.1. Patient demographics

During the 5-year study period, 2093 patients underwent appendectomy for acute appendicitis. Of the 2093 patients, 288 patients were excluded from analysis because of perforated appendicitis in preoperative diagnosis, interval appendectomy, negative appendectomy, and operation after consultation from other departments. Among the 1805 patients included for analysis, 1342 (74.3%) underwent an appendectomy within 12 hours after hospital arrival

Variables	Immediate (n = 1342)	Delayed (n = 463)	p Value
Age (years ± SD)	31.4 ± 18.2	32.8 ± 16.9	0.144
Sex			0.440
Male	761 (56.7)	253 (54.6)	
Female	581 (43.3)	210 (45.4)	
BMI (kg/m^2)	22.1 ± 4.1	22.5 ± 4.1	0.074
ASA score			0.329
1	355 (27.3)	114 (25.1)	
2	922 (70.9)	331 (72.9)	
3	18 (1.4)	7 (1.5)	
4	2 (0.2)	0 (0)	
5	2 (0.2)	2 (0.4)	
Patient interval (hours)[a]	27.8 ± 33.4	27.2 ± 44.2	0.737
WBC (10^3/dL)	13.1 ± 4.6	12.9 ± 4.2	0.495
Body temperature (°C)	36.6 ± 0.6	36.7 ± 0.5	0.001

Values are presented as number (%) unless otherwise indicated.

SD, standard deviation; BMI, body mass index; ASA, American society of anesthesiologists; WBC, white blood cell; dL, deciliter; °C, centigrade.

[a]Time from onset of symptoms to arrival at hospital.

Table 1. Patient characteristics.

(immediate group) and 463 (25.7%) underwent an appendectomy from 12 to 24 hours after hospital arrival (delayed group). No patient underwent surgery more than 24 hours after hospital arrival. Patients were on average 31.7 ± 17.9 years old and predominantly male (1014/1805, 56.2%). On average, BMI (kg/m^2) was 22.2 ± 3.9, patient interval was 27.7 ± 36.4 hours, and WBC counts (10^3/dL) were 13.0 ± 4.5. No significant differences in age, sex, BMI, ASA score, patient interval, or WBC count were noted between the two groups. Body temperature was significantly different between the immediate group (36.6 ± 0.6°C) and delayed group (36.7 ± 0.5°C) ($p = 0.001$), but was considered clinically nonsignificant because body temperatures in both groups were within the normal range (**Table 1**).

3.2. Safety-related outcomes

There were no significant differences in the laparoscopic to open conversion rate (0.5% in the immediate group and 0.2% in the delayed group), operative time (45.8 ± 21.4 minutes in the immediate group and 46.0 ± 23.6 minutes in the delayed group), perforation rate based on final pathology (12.8% in the immediate group and 12.1% in the delayed group), postoperative complication rate (6.0% in the immediate group and 6.0% in the delayed group), and readmission rate (2.5% in the immediate group and 2.2% in the delayed group) between the two groups (**Table 2**).

Variables	Immediate (n = 1342)	Delayed (n = 463)	p Value
Operative procedure			
Laparoscopy	1266 (94.3)	443 (95.7)	0.267
Open	62 (4.6)	16 (3.5)	0.288
Open conversion	7 (0.5)	1 (0.2)	0.393
Cecectomy	7 (0.5)	3 (0.6)	0.752
Operative time (minute)	45.8 ± 21.4	46.0 ± 23.6	0.833
Postoperative diagnosis			0.687
Simple	1170 (87.2)	407 (87.9)	
Perforated	172 (12.8)	56 (12.1)	
Complications			
All	80 (6.0)	28 (6.0)	0.946
Wound infection	54 (4.0)	18 (3.9)	0.897
Intra-abdominal infection	23 (1.7)	7 (1.5)	0.769
Other[a]	3 (0.2)	3 (0.6)	0.180
Readmissions	33 (2.5)	10 (2.2)	0.716

Values are presented as number (%) unless otherwise indicated.
[a]Immediate; ileus (3), delayed; obstruction (2), mesenteric lymphadenitis (1).

Table 2. Safety-related outcomes.

3.3. Economy-related outcomes

Overall length of hospital stay was significantly greater in the delayed group (3.7 ± 1.7 days) than in the immediate group (3.1 ± 1.9 days) (p = 0.000). The difference in length of postoperative hospital stay, however, was nonsignificant between the two groups (3.0 ± 1.8 days in the immediate group and 2.9 ± 1.6 days in the delayed group) (**Table 3**). Total medical cost was 2346.3 ± 735.3 US dollar in the delayed group, slightly greater than the 2257.8 ± 723.8 US dollar in the immediate group (p = 0.000).

3.4. Accuracy of radiologic modalities

The sensitivity of computed tomography (CT) (probability of patients diagnosed with nonperforated appendicitis by CT among those diagnosed with nonperforated appendicitis by pathology) was 97.0% (879/906) and specificity of CT (probability of patients diagnosed with perforated appendicitis by CT among those diagnosed with perforated appendicitis by pathology) was 46.1% (125/271) in our data (**Table 4**). The false-positive rate of CT (probability of patients diagnosed

Variables	Immediate (n = 1342)	Delayed (n = 463)	p Value
LHS (days)[a]	3.1 ± 1.9	3.7 ± 1.7	0.000
Postoperative LHS (days)	3.0 ± 1.8	2.9 ± 1.6	0.622
Cost (US dollar)	2257.8 ± 723.8	2346.3 ± 735.3	0.000

[a]LHS, length of hospital stay.

Table 3. Economy-related outcomes.

Variables	Nonperforated in pathology	Perforated in pathology	All	
Nonperforated on CT	879	146	1025	85.8%[e] (879/1025)
	97.0%[a]	53.9%[c]		
Perforated on CT	27	125	152	82.2%[f] (125/152)
	3.0%[b]	46.1%[d]		
All	906	271	1117	

Values are presented as number unless otherwise indicated.

CT, computed tomography.

[a]Sensitivity; probability of patients diagnosed with nonperforated appendicitis by CT among those diagnosed with nonperforated appendicitis by pathology.

[b]False negative rate; 1-sensitivity.

[c]False positive rate; 1-specificity.

[d]Specificity; probability of patients diagnosed with perforated appendicitis by CT among those diagnosed with perforated appendicitis by pathology.

[e]Positive predictive value; probability of patients diagnosed with nonperforated appendicitis by pathology among those diagnosed with nonperforated appendicitis by CT.

[f]Negative predictive value; probability of patients diagnosed with perforated appendicitis by pathology among those diagnosed with perforated appendicitis by CT.

Table 4. Accuracy of computed tomography.

Variables	Nonperforated in pathology	Perforated in pathology	All	
Nonperforated on US	530	58	588	90.1%[e] (530/588)
	95.5%[a]	61.1%[c]		
Perforated on US	25	37	62	59.7%[f] (37/62)
	4.5%[b]	38.9%[d]		
All	555	95	650	

Values are presented as numbers unless otherwise indicated.

US, ultrasonography.

[a]Sensitivity; probability of patients diagnosed with nonperforated appendicitis by US among those diagnosed with nonperforated appendicitis by pathology.

[b]False negative rate; 1-sensitivity.

[c]False positive rate; 1-specificity.

[d]Specificity; probability of patients diagnosed with perforated appendicitis by US among those diagnosed with perforated appendicitis by pathology.

[e]Positive predictive value; probability of patients diagnosed with nonperforated appendicitis by pathology among those diagnosed with nonperforated appendicitis by US.

[f]Negative predictive value; probability of patients diagnosed with perforated appendicitis by pathology among those diagnosed with perforated appendicitis by US.

Table 5. Accuracy of ultrasonography.

with nonperforated appendicitis by CT among those diagnosed with perforated appendicitis by pathology) was as high as 53.9% (146/271). The sensitivity of ultrasonography (US) was 95.5% (530/555) and specificity of US was 38.9% (37/95) in our records (**Table 5**). The false-positive rate of US (probability of patients diagnosed with nonperforated appendicitis by US among those diagnosed with perforated appendicitis by pathology) was as high as 61.1% (58/95).

4. Discussion

The present study demonstrated that semielective appendectomies for patients with acute nonperforated appendicitis do not increase the morbidity (defined as open conversion rate, operative time, perforation rate, postoperative complication rate, and readmission rate) but do increase economic factors such as medical costs and length of hospital stay.

Our findings were consistent with those of several other studies that have not found increased rates of complications among patients with delayed appendectomy. In a study of 380 patients with acute appendicitis, Abou-Nukta et al. [5] demonstrated that an appendectomy delay of greater than 12 hours showed no significant increase in perforation rates, operative time, or length of hospital stay. In addition, Omundsen and Dennett [8] found that there were no differences in complication rates or length of postoperative hospital stay between patients who underwent appendectomy within 12 hours and from 12 to 24 hours after admission. Omundsen and Dennett's study of 345 appendectomies only showed an increase in morbidity when appendectomy was delayed more than 24 hours. Surana et al. [6] reported no difference in complication rates between patients undergoing appendectomy within 6 hours compared to 6 to 18 hours after admission in a study of 695 children with appendicitis. In a similar study of 126 pediatric patients with acute non-perforated appendicitis, Yardeni et al. [7] demonstrated that there were no significant increases in the complication rates or perforation rates when appendectomies were performed within 6, 6 to 12, or more than 12 hours after admission. In a population-based study that used a database of 32,782 patients and was the largest study supporting this semi-elective approach, Ingraham et al. [4] found that a delay in appendectomy was not associated with increased 30-day morbidity.

In contrast to these studies, several others continue to support the current standard of appendectomy as a standard emergency procedure. In 1081 adult patients with acute appendicitis, Ditillo et al. [9] found that the risk of developing advanced pathology and complications increased with time until appropriate treatments, suggesting that a delay in appendectomy was unsafe. Udgiri et al. [10] reported that the complication rates, lengths of hospital stay, and readmissions were greater in a delayed appendectomy group (performed more than 10 hours after admission) than in an immediate appendectomy group (performed less than 10 hours after admission) in a study of 211 patients with appendicitis. Recently, Teixeira et al. [11] showed that while an appendectomy delay of more than 6 hours did not increase the risk of perforation, it significantly increased the risk of surgical site infection in 4529 patients with nonperforated appendicitis. In contrast, the present study showed no difference in surgical site infection rate, which was approximately 5% in each group.

The safety of delayed appendectomy can be explained by the development of medical technologies, particularly the injection of antibiotics to halt the progression of appendicitis. A number of studies have shown the effectiveness of antibiotics in treating perforated appendicitis [12–14]. In most cases, antibiotic administration leads to resolution of the infectious and inflammatory processes of perforated appendicitis, which allows elective appendectomy to be performed 6–8 weeks after the initial presentation of disease. Moreover, two randomized controlled trials suggested that acute appendicitis could be successfully treated with antibiotics and that antibiotics might be a first-line therapy in acute appendicitis [2, 3].

Nowadays, we just give one injection of antibiotics just before surgery. In the case of severe wound complications, we have used antibiotics even if it did not follow guidelines.

Among a total of 1805 cases, we performed 190 appendectomies (10.5%) for acute appendicitis between the hours of 11 PM and 8 AM. When a patient was diagnosed with nonperforated appendicitis at these hours, we often had no choice but to delay an operation, offer antibiotic therapy, and schedule an operation for the following day. The unavailability of an emergency operating room or operating team members such as an anesthesiologist, nurse, or assistant prohibited the prompt operation. The results of this report may lessen surgeons' stress in this situation, as the increasing risk of perforation and subsequent morbidity in appendicitis progression may be less significant than previously thought. This optimistic finding could have a positive psychological effect on surgeons, resulting in a more meticulous operation the following day with enhanced care for patients. In addition, the current government policy that surgical specialists should care for their patients in the emergency room greatly increases the responsibility of surgeons. Our findings suggest that surgeons could delay operations for less critically ill patients, such as those with nonperforated appendicitis, in order to appropriately care for those requiring immediate attention, such as trauma patients and critical care patients, especially in situations with limited staff.

Accurate preoperative diagnosis to clarify whether the appendix is perforated or not must be a prerequisite to delayed appendectomy. CT is a main diagnostic tool with high sensitivity and specificity for acute appendicitis. The routine use of CT in patients with suspected acute appendicitis has been shown to shorten the time to operating room admission, reduce the number of negative appendectomies, and reduce medical costs [15]. Ultrasonography is another useful modality commonly used for children, pregnant patients, and outpatients, because it is noninvasive, does not require patient preparation, and avoids unnecessary exposure to ionizing radiation. Moreover, Peña et al. [16] demonstrated that an imaging protocol using US and CT was useful for distinguishing between nonperforated and perforated appendicitis, as shown by a marked decrease in the perforation and negative appendectomy rates in 1338 children with suspected appendicitis. However, this study showed that the false-positive rate of CT and US was as high as 53.9% (146/271) and 61.1% (58/95), respectively. As radiologic readings are not infallible, surgeons need to confirm the presence of perforation using symptoms, physical examinations, and laboratory findings. Radiologists must also pay close, critical attention to their radiologic interpretations. In our data, there were false positive and negative findings in CT and U/S. But there is no perfect diagnostic modality established of appendicitis before surgery. This was one of the limitations of our study.

At the beginning of this study, we predicted that there would be little difference in medical costs between the two groups because the additional hospitalization fees for the delayed group might be similar to the additional nighttime surgery fees for the immediate group. However, medical costs were significantly increased for the delayed group because the additional hospitalization fees were more expensive than the additional nighttime surgery fees in the immediate group. Surgeons should consider that increased medical costs can be a burden for patients and health insurance companies. In addition, the emotional and unanticipated economic cost of extended hospital stays in the delayed group should not be dismissed.

In conclusion, delayed appendectomy is safe for patients with acute nonperforated appendicitis. It can improve quality of provided care from surgeons, enhance quality of care for patients, and increase effective utilization of medical resources and operating rooms for life-threatening emergencies.

Author details

Sung Il Choi[1,2*]

*Address all correspondence to: drchoi@khu.ac.kr

1 Department of Surgery, Kyung Hee University School of Medicine, Kyung Hee University Hospital at Gangdong, Seoul, Korea

2 Department of Surgery, Kyung Hee University School of Medicine, Kyung Hee University Hospital, Seoul, Korea

References

[1] Berry Jr J, Malt RA. Appendicitis near its centenary. Annals of Surgery. Nov 1984;**200**(5): 567-575

[2] Hansson J, Körner U, Khorram-Manesh A, Solberg A, Lundholm K. Randomized clinical trial of antibiotic therapy versus appendicectomy as primary treatment of acute appendicitis in unselected patients. The British Journal of Surgery. May 2009;**96**(5):473-481. DOI: 10.1002/bjs.6482

[3] Styrud J, Eriksson S, Nilsson I, Ahlberg G, Haapaniemi S, Neovius G, et al. Appendectomy versus antibiotic treatment in acute appendicitis. A prospective multicenter randomized controlled trial. World Journal of Surgery. Jun 2006;**30**(6):1033-1037

[4] Ingraham AM, Cohen ME, Bilimoria KY, Ko CY, Hall BL, Russell TR, et al. Effect of delay to operation on outcomes in adults with acute appendicitis. Archives of Surgery. Sep 2010;**145**(9):886-892. DOI: 10.1001/archsurg.2010.184

[5] Abou-Nukta F, Bakhos C, Arroyo K, Koo Y, Martin J, Reinhold R, et al. Effects of delaying appendectomy for acute appendicitis for 12 to 24 hours. Archives of Surgery. May 2006;**141**(5):504-506. discussioin 506-7

[6] Surana R, Quinn F, Puri P. Is it necessary to perform appendicectomy in the middle of the night in children? British Medical Journal. May 1, 1993;**306**(6886):1168

[7] Yardeni D, Hirschl RB, Drongowski RA, Teitelbaum DH, Geiger JD, Coran AG. Delayed versus immediate surgery in acute appendicitis: Do we need to operate during the night? Journal of Pediatric Surgery. Mar 2004;**39**(3):464-469 (discussion 464-469)

[8] Omundsen M, Dennett E. Delay to appendicectomy and associated morbidity: A retrospective review. ANZ Journal of Surgery. Mar 2006;**76**(3):153-155

[9] Ditillo MF, Dziura JD, Rabinovici R. Is it safe to delay appendectomy in adults with acute appendicitis? Annals of Surgery. Nov 2006;**244**(5):656-660

[10] Udgiri N, Curras E, Kella VK, Nagpal K, Cosgrove J. Appendicitis, is it an emergency? The American Surgeon. Jul 2011;**77**(7):898-901

[11] Teixeira PG, Sivrikoz E, Inaba K, Talving P, Lam L, Demetriades D. Appendectomy timing: Waiting until the next morning increases the risk of surgical site infections. Annals of Surgery. Sep 2012;**256**(3):538-543. DOI: 10.1097/SLA.0b013e318265ea13

[12] Bufo AJ, Shah RS, Li MH, Cyr NA, Hollabaugh RS, Hixson SD, et al. Interval appendectomy for perforated appendicitis in children. Journal of Laparoendoscopic & Advanced Surgical Techniques. Part A. Aug 1998;**8**(4):209-214

[13] Weiner DJ, Katz A, Hirschl RB, Drongowski R, Coran AG. Interval appendectomy in perforated appendicitis. Pediatric Surgery International. Feb 1995;**10**(2-3):82-85

[14] Mazziotti M, Marley E, Winthrop A, Fitzgerald P, Walton M, Langer J. Histopathologic analysis of interval appendectomy specimens: Support for the role of interval appendectomy. Journal of Pediatric Surgery. Jun 1997;**32**(6):806-809

[15] Rao PM, Rhea JT, Novelline RA, Mostafavi AA, McCabe CJ. Effect of computed tomography of the appendix on treatment of patients and use of hospital resources. The New England Journal of Medicine. Jan 15, 1998;**338**(3):141-146

[16] Peña BMG, Taylor GA, Fishman SJ, Mandl KD. Effect of an imaging protocol on clinical outcomes among pediatric patients with appendicitis. Pediatrics. Dec 2002;**110**(6):1088-1093

Section 3

Acute Appendicitis in Children

Chapter 6

Management of Pediatric Appendicitis

Volkan Sarper Erikci

Additional information is available at the end of the chapter

http://dx.doi.org/10.5772/intechopen.72793

Abstract

Appendicitis is the most common surgical diagnosis for children who present with abdominal pain to the emergency department. However, there are nonspecific examination findings and variable historical features during its presentation. Diagnosis of appendicitis in the pediatric patient may be challenging for the clinician dealing with these children. It is important to have a high index of suspicion and taking a detailed history and physical examination. In diagnosis of appendicitis, adjunctive studies that may be useful are the white blood cell count, C-reactive protein, urinalysis, ultrasonography and computerized tomography when necessary. When appendicitis is suspected, patients should receive immediate surgical consultation, as well as volume replacement and antibiotics if indicated. The most accurate diagnostic tool is perhaps the serial examinations by the same examiner. With this timely approach, it will be possible to prevent the significant morbidity that is associated with delayed diagnoses in younger patients.

Keywords: appendicitis, children, management

1. Introduction

Acute appendicitis is the most common surgical emergency in children and adolescents. Although uncommon in preschool children, it may be present at any age. The lifetime risk of developing appendicitis is 7–8%, with a peak incidence in the teenage years [1]. There are 250,000 cases in the USA annually and the majority occurs in children with the ages between 6 and 10 years. Nearly one-third of children with appendicitis have perforation at the time of surgical treatment. It affects males more frequently than females with male predominance (M:F ratio 3:2). There is a seasonal variation in the occurrence of appendicitis so that its presentation is increased in the summer months with perforated appendicitis occurring more frequently in the fall and winter seasons [2]. Despite advances and innovations in fluid

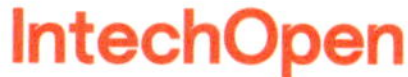

resuscitation and antibiotics, appendicitis especially in preschool children may be difficult to diagnose and is still associated with significant morbidity even mortality.

2. Embryology and anatomy

As a continuation of the inferior tip of the cecum that becomes visible during the eighth week of gestation, appendix rotates to its final position which is the posteromedial aspect of cecum. According to Treves, there are several variations that can be classified into four types: Type 1, the appendix is of fetal type with a funnel shape; Type 2, the appendix originates from the cecal fundus; Type 3, the appendix originates dorsomedially out of the cecum (most common type); and Type 4, the appendix originates directly beside the ileal orifice [3].

The position of the appendix varies among individuals. According to a study comprising 10,000 cases, 5 positions can be identified: ascending appendix in the retrocecal recess in 65% of cases (most common), descending appendix in the iliac fossa in 31% of cases, transverse appendix in the retrocecal recess in 2.5% of cases, paracecal and preileal ascending appendix in 1% of cases and paracecal and postileal ascending appendix in 0.5% of cases [4]. During surgical treatment, it is important to distinguish if the appendix is non-fixed (appendix libera) or fixed (appendix fixa).

With an average length of 8 cm, the size of appendix varies from 0.3 to 33 cm and its diameter of ranges from 5 to 10 mm. The blood comes from appendiceal branch of the ileocolic artery. There are a few submucosal lymph follicles present at birth and they increase to nearly 200 by the age of 12 and the number of these lymph follicles decreases after the age of 30.

3. Etiology and pathogenesis

Obstruction of the appendiceal lumen is usually the first factor that starts the illness. If unresolved, this obstruction leads to vascular congestion, ischemic necrosis and subsequent infection. Inspissated fecal material or a fecalith are the most common causes that lead to appendiceal luminal obstruction. Other causes of obstruction include lymphoid follicle hyperplasia, foreign bodies, carcinoid or other tumors and rarely parasites. Fecaliths are found in approximately 40% cases of acute appendicitis, 65% cases of gangrenous appendicitis and approximately 90% cases of perforated appendicitis [5].

As the appendiceal mucosa continues to secrete the mucus after occlusion of the appendix lumen, this leads to a rapid increase of intraluminal pressure. Secretion of as little as 0.5 mL leads to an increase of pressure of approximately 45 mm Hg, according to the law of Laplace [5]. This phenomenon also explains the rapid perforation of appendix within a few hours of inflammation. For this reason, all the patients with suspected acute appendicitis, need hospitalization and close clinical monitoring if appendectomy is not to be performed immediately.

Distention stimulates nerve endings of visceral afferent pain fibers and leads to a dull, diffuse mid-abdominal pain that cannot be easily located by the children. As the distention increases, it causes reflex nausea and vomiting and once the inflammatory process has involved the serosal part of the appendix and parietal peritoneum, the characteristic finding of shift of the pain from periumbilical area to the right lower abdominal quadrant occurs. Impaired blood supply leads to compromise of the appendiceal mucosa allowing bacterial invasion of the deeper locations. Absorption of bacterial toxins and necrotic material causes fever, tachycardia and leukocytosis. As the pressure increases, finally perforation occurs usually through the infarcted areas. Although in some patients, the disease may spontaneously resolve, untreated obstruction of the appendiceal lumen usually leads to gangrene and perforation.

4. Clinical presentation

Although appendicitis can affect any age group, it is extremely rare in neonates and infants. It is well known that the clinic of appendicitis in infants is different from older children. Indeed, appendicitis in infants is more violent, extremely dangerous and associated with the clinic of severe intoxication, which is due to the growing phenomena of peritonitis. Defense mechanisms such as inability to limit the inflammation process, decreased amount of omentum in infants, are also important factors that make infants unprotected against the ongoing inflammation process. Older children present clinical signs and symptoms which are quite variable in pattern and order of appearance. As a first symptom, pain usually begins as a dull and vague pattern at the periumbilical area but with time, it may localize to the right lower quadrant. *To be precise, Charles McBurney himself in 1889, localized the pain in the following way: "I affirm that in each case the most severe pain due to finger pressure is exactly localized at a distance of 1.5-2 inches from the anterior superior iliac spine, on the line, conducted from this iliac spine to the navel."* Children usually report a gradual increase in pain intensity as the disease progresses. The anatomical variability in the locations of appendix vermiformis (i.e., retrocecal, pelvic, preileal) is common and may alter pain symptoms accordingly. Pelvic or retrocecal appendicitis may be only present with right lower quadrant pain without periumbilical pain. Flank pain and referred testicular pain are also common symptoms in children with pelvic or retrocecal appendicitis. If the inflamed appendix has a close relationship with ureter or bladder, it may produce symptoms associated with urinary tractus such as urinary frequency, dysuria, urinary retention and bladder distention. It is traditionally known that severe gastrointestinal symptoms that develop prior to the onset of pain usually indicate a diagnosis other than acute appendicitis. On the other hand, mild gastrointestinal symptoms such as decreased appetite, indigestion and changes in bowel habits may develop within a few hours of pain onset.

Typically patients with uncomplicated appendicitis have low-grade fever. Fever above 38.6 degrees, tachycardia and leukocytosis develop as a consequence of mediators released by ischemic tissues, white blood cells and bacteria. Children with appendicitis avoid movement and tend to lie in bed with their knees flexed. Hyperesthesia of the skin can be elicited by touching the skin of the patient. Abdominal tenderness associated with appendicitis varies with the stage of the disease and location of the inflamed vermiform appendix. Classical "McBurney's point" that is the area one-third the distance from anterior superior iliac spine to the umbilicus, is the most common site of maximal tenderness that is found on the abdominal

Gastrointestinal causes-liver, spleen and biliary tract disorders

Gastroenteritis

Mesenteric lymphadenitis

Constipation

Trauma

Peptic ulcer disease

Meckel's diverticulum

Inflammatory bowel disease

Cholecystitis

Intussusception

Neoplasm (carcinoid, lymphoma)

Food poisoning

Intestinal obstruction

Omental torsion

Pancreatitis

Volvulus

Diverticulitis

Perforated viscus

Hepatitis

Cholecystitis

Splenic infarction and splenic rupture

Genitourinary causes

Urinary tract infection

Urinary calculi

Pyelonephritis

Pelvic inflammatory disease

Ectopic pregnancy

Ovarian/testicular torsion

Hematocolpos

Endometriosis

Mittelschmerz

Tubo-ovarian abscess

Ovarian cyst rupture

Metabolic disorders

Diabetic ketoacidosis
Hypoglycemia
Porphyria
Acute adrenal insufficiency
Hematologic disorders
Sickle cell disease
Henoch-Schönlein purpura
Hemolytic uremic syndrome
Pulmonary causes
Pneumonia (right lobe basilar)
Pleuritis
Pulmonary infarction
Drugs and toxins
Erythromycin
Salicylates
Lead poisoning
Other causes
Familial Mediterranean fever
Infantile colic
Parasitic infection
Psoas abscess
Functional pain
Angioneurotic edema

Table 1. Differential diagnosis of pediatric appendicitis.

wall. Rectal tenderness may be observed in patients with pelvic appendicitis. In the case of malrotation, the tenderness due to appendicitis may occur on unusual locations which may be away from the usual site.

There are some clinical signs that should produce high index of suspicion of appendicitis, namely "Rovsings' sign" (palpation of left lower quadrant producing tenderness over the right iliac fossa), and it is a reliable indicator of appendicitis in childhood. The "psoas sign" that is commonly observed in retrocecal appendicitis and the "obturator sign" suggesting pelvic appendicitis are the other useful clinical signs that should prompt clinician to diagnose acute appendicitis early. The physical examination of a patient suspected to have appendicitis (especially pelvic appendicitis) is missing without rectal exam which may reveal a tender palpable mass or abscess.

Differential diagnosis of acute appendicitis has a wide spectrum of diseases and includes gastroenteritis, inflammatory bowel disease such as Crohn's disease, cholelithiasis, mesenteric adenitis, pancreatitis, peptic ulcer disease, Meckel's diverticulitis, constipation, intussusception and many other disease states (**Table 1**). Systemic diseases including diabetic ketoacidosis, lupus erythematosus, hemolytic uremic syndrome, sickle cell crisis, Henoch-Schönlein purpura and parasitic infections may produce symptoms suggesting acute appendicitis. In females with certain situations such as ectopic pregnancy, ovarian torsion, developmental ovarian cysts and pelvic inflammatory disease, a misdiagnosis of acute appendicitis may cause unnecessary surgical interventions. Pneumonia, particularly affecting the right lower lobe of lung, urinary tract diseases such as renal or ureteric stones, pyelonephritis and urinary tract infections can also mimic acute appendicitis. Children with cystic fibrosis have a higher incidence of acute appendicitis. A neonate with appendicitis should increase the suspicion of Hirschsprung's disease in the mind of the clinician.

5. Diagnosis

History and physical examination is important in diagnosing appendicitis in children. The most accurate diagnostic tool is perhaps the serial examinations by the same examiner while the child is cooperative with the clinician. Before starting the palpation of the abdomen, the child should be asked to point out the location of the abdominal pain. Cutaneous hyperesthesia is often an early finding derived from the T10 to L1 nerve roots. There is a mild abdominal pain that cannot be localized at the early stages of the disease. As the disease progresses, localized tenderness is most often found at the McBurney's point. Rectal tenderness may be observed in pelvic appendicitis and tenderness midway between the 12th rib and the posterior superior iliac spine is detected in patients with retrocecal appendicitis. If malrotation accompanies the disease, position of the inflamed appendix has a role in the changing locations of tenderness. Peritonitis ensues as the disease progresses to perforation with generalized abdominal rigidity. Rebound tenderness is seldom necessary for diagnosis and is usually regarded as an unnecessary discomfort for children. Routine rectal examination in diagnosing appendicitis in childhood is a matter of debate and if other signs suggest to the diagnosis of appendicitis, rectal examination may be unnecessary. But it is especially helpful diagnostic tool for patients with pelvic appendicitis with abscess or those with uterine or adnexal pathologic conditions. It should be re-emphasized that when the diagnosis is unclear, with the aid of serial physical examinations, it is possible to decrease the number of unnecessary surgical interventions that may increase risk to the patient if performed. This issue is very important, because in a recent study, among the children undergoing appendectomy, 6.3% in Canada and 4.3% in the USA, are subsequently found to have a normal appendix and it has been reported that a misdiagnosis of appendicitis that leads to negative appendectomy ranges up to 30% [6].

The most often used laboratory aids to diagnose appendicitis are white blood cell (WBC) count, absolute neutrophil count (ANC) and C-reactive protein (CRP) but these tests alone are not helpful or predictive. Leukocyte count above 10,000 is observed in greater than 90% of children with acute appendicitis. But normal WBC count may also be observed in 5% of patients with appendicitis. A shift to left is a usual finding and is of better diagnostic value compared to ANC. A neutrophil-lymphocyte ratio of greater than 3.5 has a greater specificity and sensitivity in diagnosing appendicitis.

There are numerous appendicitis scoring systems that have been suggested as an adjunct to diagnosis of appendicitis. Two systems, namely the Alvarado score and the Pediatric Appendicitis Score (PAS), have been extensively studied but do not have 100% sensitivity and specificity in the diagnosis of appendicitis and they do not replace an experienced pediatric surgeon [7–9]. It has been documented that a pediatric surgeon can differentiate appendicitis from other abdominal disorders with 92% accuracy [10]. Urinalysis is helpful in differentiating urinary tract infections and urolithiasis from appendicitis. However, when inflamed appendix is in close proximity with ureter, hematuria and pyuria may also be detected even if there is no urinary tract infection or urolithiasis.

Imaging studies may be useful in cases where the diagnosis is equivocal and plain film radiography may have a value. The incidence of presence of a fecalith that can be seen on direct roentgenograms ranges from 10 to 20% of cases with appendicitis and this ratio increases accordingly in patients with complicated appendicitis. Other subtle plain film findings are sentinel loop in the right lower quadrant, lumbar scoliosis with a concavity to the right lower quadrant, mass effect due to pelvic abscess, loss of psoas shadow and obliteration of the properitoneal fat stripe. It is necessary to have a chest radiograph for ruling out right lower lobe pneumonia. Although it is usually useful tool in the management of children with intussusception, barium enema may rarely be performed in children suspected of having appendicitis. Barium enema findings in appendicitis include: incomplete filling of the appendix, extrinsic mass effect on the cecum or terminal ileum and irregularities of the appendiceal lumen.

With a sensitivity of 85% and specificity of greater than 90%, ultrasonography (US) is a useful diagnostic tool if performed especially by skilled hands. Sonographic criteria for the diagnosis of appendicitis is demonstration of a noncompressible appendix that is 7 mm or larger in diameter, a wall thicker than 2 mm or an irregular wall that is rigid, and lacks peristalsis [11]. Other findings that may be helpful in diagnosing appendicitis include absence of air in the appendiceal lumen, periappendiceal fat changes, visible appendicolith, complex mass, mesenteric lymph nodes and free fluid [11]. Advantages of US include lack of sedation, contrast agents and radiation during procedure [12]. On the other hand, there are also disadvantages regarding US that include need for operator experience, a lack of regular availability during off hours, difficult visualization especially in obese children [13]. Computed tomography (CT) is also useful for inconclusive cases. It combines the advantages of many other imaging modalities, including rapid acquisition time and a lack of operator dependency [14]. The findings of an enlarged appendix (>6 mm), appendiceal wall thickening (>1 mm) and appendiceal wall enhancement are useful diagnostic criteria that are found in CT. Comparing US and CT in diagnosing appendicitis in children, it has been proposed that US is more specific and CT is more sensitive [15]. Magnetic resonance imaging (MRI) has a high diagnostic accuracy for appendicitis, but it has certain disadvantages including limited utility, lack of availability in many centers, lengthy acquisition time, need for sedation or anesthesia and high cost compared to other imaging modalities [15]. It should be re-emphasized again that these radiological diagnostic modalities, if used routinely, cause hospital resource utilization and delay in surgical treatment. Besides, potential cancer risk associated with ionizing radiation from CT should also be kept in mind and these imaging tools should be reserved for patients with uncertain findings related to appendicitis.

Laparoscopy may be a useful diagnostic tool for patients with inconclusive findings related to appendicitis. It may be a helpful diagnostic aid especially in obese and overweight children. Laparoscopy should be kept in mind when other diagnostic modalities are not enough for diagnosing appendicitis and the attending surgeon should not hesitate to perform laparoscopy.

6. Treatment

There are several treatment modalities of appendicitis with a wide spectrum ranging from nonoperative management to open or laparoscopic surgical interventions. Nonoperative management of appendicitis has been an interest for many scientists and several trials demonstrated successful nonoperative management of acute appendicitis in 70– 85% of cases in the one-year follow-up [16, 17]. On the other hand, it has been stated in another meta-analysis that the combined failure and recurrence rates in nonoperative patients made this approach less effective overall [18]. Regarding the nonoperative management of pediatric appendicitis, children revealed a success rate ranging from 75 to 80%, and in a recent study, up to 89% success rate of nonoperative management has been reported [19, 20]. It has also been demonstrated that as compared to surgically treated patients, nonoperative patients reported higher quality-of-life scores at 30 days [20]. In some situations, nonoperative management of appendicitis may be unsuccessful and one of these predictors of failure of nonoperative management has been reported to be presence of appendicolith on imaging studies [21]. Another study on the nonoperative management of uncomplicated appendicitis demonstrated a failure rate of 60% and was halted early [22]. To sum up, although there are no consensus in which patients should receive nonoperative treatment, it should be emphasized that nonoperative management is permissible only with uncomplicated acute appendicitis for carefully selected children and it is possible and should be kept in mind.

In the surgical management of appendicitis, the goals are to minimize complications and cost, decrease patient anxiety and improve quality of life. Although according to the traditional thinking that emergent appendectomy should be performed at the time of diagnosis, immediate surgical intervention is not considered mandatory for most patients. Many centers dealing with pediatric appendicitis now perform appendectomies in the day time for patients presenting at night time [23]. With this approach, the stress that occurs in the overnight appendectomies for both children, their families and surgeon is avoided. Besides, complication and perforation rates are similar for patients undergoing surgery within 6 hours of admission compared to those undergoing surgery between 6 and 16 hours after admission to the hospital. The majority of pediatric surgeons perform appendectomy within 8 hours after admission. It should be emphasized that the delay in the emergency operation is permissible only with uncomplicated acute appendicitis and after an expedient resuscitation, all the patients with appendicitis must undergo timely surgical exploration.

Initial therapy starts with intravenous fluid resuscitation, broad spectrum antibiotic coverage and keeping the patient nothing per mouth. There is a trend toward decreasing the duration of antibiotic therapy. The recommended duration of antibiotic therapy is preoperative plus 24 hours postoperative period for simple appendicitis and a 10-day course of ampicillin, gentamicin and metronidazole or clindamycin for complicated appendicitis, and these therapies are known as gold standard. On the other hand, it has been documented that both piperacillin/tazobactam and cefoxitin have been shown to be at least as effective as the triple-drug regimen and may also decrease the length of hospital stay and costs [24]. Nevertheless, total length of antibiotic therapy should be determined by the clinical condition of the patient (resolution of fever, pain, bowel function) and WBC count [25].

Surgical treatment modalities include open technique and laparoscopic appendectomy. Except for specific situations including any surgical intervention having right lower quadrant incision such as Meckel's diverticulectomy or intussusception reduction, incidental appendectomy is no longer performed routinely and does not have any benefit. The first appendectomy for acute appendicitis was performed by a British surgeon Lawson Tait in 1880. He removed the gangrenous appendix in a 17-year-old girl. Charles McBurney in 1894 described the muscle splitting incision. In his description, a transverse or oblique right lower quadrant incision is performed and by splitting the muscles, abdominal cavity is entered and mesoappendix is divided followed by excision of the appendix at its base [26]. There are different techniques of management of appendiceal stump including simple ligation, ligation and inversion using a purse-string, or a pure inversion without ligature. The choice of stump management directly relates to attending surgeon.

The world's first complete laparoscopic appendectomy with a stitched mesentery and immersion of stump in the wall of the cecum and Z-stitches was performed in 1981 by the pioneer in minimally invasive surgery, a German gynecologist Kurt Semm. It should be noted that as a gynecologist, he performed only a passing appendectomy for endometriosis of the appendix or chronic appendicitis. Since this first description of endoscopic appendectomy, laparoscopic appendectomies are being performed more and more commonly nowadays and today laparoscopic appendectomies have largely replaced the open surgery by up to 91% [27]. There are several different operative approaches in the laparoscopic management of appendicitis including three-port laparoscopic intervention, transumbilical laparoscopic appendectomy, and single-port/incision techniques. Advantages of laparoscopy include shorter hospital stay, decreased postoperative pain and wound complications, ability to diagnose inconclusive cases, surgical ease in obese patients and faster recovery after surgery. On the other hand, there are disadvantages of laparoscopic approach which are a higher cost of equipment, longer operative time, time needed for learning curve in laparoscopy education, experience required for surgeons and increased incidence of intra-abdominal infection. It has been previously stated that complication rates are lower compared to open appendectomy except that the postoperative intra-abdominal abscess rate is higher with laparoscopic approach [28]. But this topic seems to be changed as it has been found in the meta-analysis and multi-institutional reviews that there are no differences in intra-abdominal abscess rates following laparoscopic surgery compared to open surgical interventions for appendicitis [29, 30]. To sum up, laparoscopy is a safe and effective means of performing an appendectomy in the treatment of pediatric appendicitis.

If a normal appendix is found at laparotomy (5–15% of cases), the abdomen is systematically inspected for evidence of inflammatory bowel disease, a Meckel's diverticulum, mesenteric adenitis and peptic ulcer disease. In females, fallopian tubes and ovaries should be identified and inspected for ovarian cysts or torsion, and for rare occurrence of isolated tubal torsion and pelvic inflammatory disease. Following open surgery or laparoscopic approach, there comes the question of drain usage. Although it has long been stated that irrigating the abdominal cavity is not recommended in patients with simple appendicitis and may have a role in the management of complicated appendicitis, previous studies demonstrated that there was no favoring irrigation for peritoneal contamination in perforated appendicitis [31]. Even an increase in abscesses resulting from the use of irrigation compared to no irrigation following laparoscopic surgical intervention has been reported [32].

Management of children with a palpable abdominal mass who present late (i.e., several days or weeks) is another controversial topic. Some suggest an immediate appendectomy whereas others perform the procedure only when a mass is confirmed either as a result of radiological diagnostic work-up or during the surgery with the patient under anesthesia. In a meta-analysis, evaluating early versus delayed appendectomy for perforated appendicitis concluded that delayed operation was associated with significantly less overall complications, wound infections, intra-abdominal abscesses, bowel obstructions and reoperations [33]. On the other hand, early appendectomy, compared to interval appendectomy, significantly reduced the time away from normal activities [33]. Opponents to interval appendectomy suggest that it is unnecessary because only 14% of patients have recurrent symptoms, and after initial diagnosis, recurrence is uncommon within 2 years. Nevertheless, it is very important that if an operation is to be performed, great care should be taken to avoid damage to adjacent structures such as small intestine, the fallopian tubes, ovaries and ureters. In the case of well-localized periappendiceal abscess or phlegmon, after a prolonged antibiotic therapy (2–3 weeks) CT or sonographic-guided percutaneous abscess drainage may be another option in the treatment of these children. The current standard for patients presenting with a palpable abdominal mass who are usually young children with perforation, is conservative management with interval appendectomy after 8–12 weeks.

7. Complications

Complication rates after appendectomy differ greatly with regard to the severity of the appendicitis. Complications are rarely seen after simple appendicitis but are more often seen in children with complicated appendicitis. Wound infection is the most common complication after appendectomy. With the worldwide usage of antibiotics, the rate of wound infection has fallen from 50% to less than 5%, even in complicated appendicitis. Other complications of appendicitis include intra-abdominal abscess formation, wound dehiscence, postoperative intestinal obstruction, prolonged ileus and rarely enterocutaneous fistula. It has been reported that the postoperative risk of an intra-abdominal abscess is approximately 20% for children with perforated appendicitis, and the risk for children with simple appendicitis to develop an abscess is less than 0.8% [31]. Tubal infertility and pylephlebitis may also be observed after surgical treatment for complicated appendicitis such as pelvic and subhepatic appendicitis, respectively. Sepsis and multisystem organ failure can occur in young children with a prolonged illness before definite diagnosis. As the antibiotics have markedly decreased the incidence of infectious complications, the mortality rate for complicated appendicitis has dropped dramatically to nearly zero. The overall morbidity in children with complicated appendicitis is less than 10%.

8. Conclusion

Appendicitis occurs most commonly between the ages of 10 and 11 years. The classical signs and symptoms of migrating pain to the right lower quadrant and rebound tenderness are present in less than half of the children presenting with appendicitis. When the diagnosis is certain, the combination of evaluation and prompt surgical intervention is all that is needed. If the diagnosis of appendicitis is inconclusive, a period of observation including usage of scoring systems for evaluating the patient followed by radiological imaging modalities becomes a matter of necessity rather than of choice. As CT scans increase radiation exposure, US should be the choice of imaging modality in these patients. Laparoscopic approaches now constitute more than 90% of appendectomies in these patients even in cases with perforated appendicitis. In selected cases, appendicitis can be managed nonoperatively. Although provided that care is given by experienced clinicians and institutions, the best outcome for children with appendicitis may be anticipated, a small number of patients may still develop complications following surgical treatment of appendicitis. Nevertheless, the long-term outcome for the majority of children who undergo appendectomy is very good.

Author details

Volkan Sarper Erikci

Address all correspondence to: verikci@yahoo.com

Department of Pediatric Surgery, Saglık Bilimleri University, İzmir Tepecik Training Hospital, Izmir, Turkey

References

[1] Addis DG, Shaffer N, Fowler BS, et al. The epidemiology of appendicitis and appendectomy in the United States. American Journal of Epidemiology. 1990;**132**(5):910-925

[2] Deng Y, Chang DC, Zhang Y, et al. Seasonal and day of the week variations of perforated appendicitis in US children. Pediatric Surgery International. 2010;**26**(7):691-696

[3] Treves F. Lectures on the anatomy of the intestinal canal and peritoneum in man. British Medical Journal. 1885;**1**(415):527-580

[4] Wakeley CPG. Position of the vermiform appendix as ascertained by analysis of 10,000 cases. Journal of Anatomy. 1933;**67**:277

[5] Arnbjornsson E, Bengmark S. Obstruction of the appendix lumen in relation to pathogenesis of acute appendicitis. Acta Chirurgica Scandinavica. 1985;**42**:184

[6] Cheong LH, Emil S. Outcomes of pediatric appendicitis: An international comparison of the United States and Canada. JAMA Surgery. 2014;**149**(1):50-55

[7] Escriba A, Gamell AM, Fernandez Y, et al. Prospective validation of two systems of classification for the diagnosis of acute appendicitis. Pediatric Emergency Care. 2011; **27**:165-169

[8] Rezak A, Abbas H, Ajemian MS, et al. Decreased use of computed tomography with a modified scoring system in the diagnosis of pediatric acute appendicitis. Archives of Surgery. 2011;**146**:64-67

[9] Goldman RD, Carter S, Stephens S. Prospective validation of the pediatric appendicitis score. The Journal of Pediatrics. 2008;**153**:278-282

[10] Williams RF, Blakely M, Fischer PE, et al. Diagnosing ruptured appendicitis preoperatively in pediatric patients. Journal of the American College of Surgeons. 2009; **208**(5):819-825

[11] Schupp CJ, Klingmuller V, Strauch K, et al. Typical signs of acute appendicitis in ultrasonography mimicked by other disease? Pediatric Surgery International. 2010;**26**:697-702

[12] Binkovitz LA, Unsdorfer KML, Thapa P, et al. Pediatric appendiceal ultrasound accuracy, determinacy and clinical outcomes. Pediatric Radiology. 2015;**45**(13):1934-1944

[13] Yiğiter M, Kantarcı M, Yalçın O, et al. Does obesity limit the sonographic diagnosis of appendicitis in children? Journal of Clinical Ultrasound. 2010;**39**(4):187-190

[14] Bachur RG, Dayan PS, Bajaj L, et al. The effect of abdominal pain duration on the accuracy of diagnostic imaging for pediatric appendicitis. Annals of Emergency Medicine. 2012; **60**(5):582-590.e3

[15] Kulaylat AN, Moore MM, Engbrecht BW, et al. An implemented MRI program to eliminate radiation from the evaluation of pediatric appendicitis. Journal of Pediatric Surgery. 2015;**50**(8):1359-1363

[16] Di SS, Sibilio A, Giorgini E, et al. The NOTA study (non operative treatment for acute appendicitis): Prospective study on the efficacy and safety of antibiotics (amoxicillin and clavulanic acid) for treating patients with right lower quadrant abdominal pain and long-term follow-up of conservatively treated suspected appendicitis. Annals of Surgery. 2014;**260**(1):109-117

[17] Salminen P, Paajanen H, Rautio T, et al. Antibiotic therapy vs appendectomy for treatment of uncomplicated acute appendicitis: The APPAC randomized clinical trial. Journal of the American Medical Association. 2015;**313**(23):2340-2348

[18] Mason RJ, Moazzez A, Sohn H, et al. Meta-analysis of randomized trials comparing antibiotic therapy with appendectomy for acute uncomplicated (no abscess or phlegmon) appendicitis. Surgical Infections. 2012;**13**(2):74-84

[19] Hartwich J, Luks FI, Watson-Smith D, et al. Nonoperative treatment of acute appendicitis in children: A feasibility study. Journal of Pediatric Surgery. 2016;**51**(1):111-116

[20] Minecci PC, Mahida JB, Lodwick DL, et al. Effectiveness of patient choice in nonoperative vs surgical management of pediatric uncomplicated acute appendicitis. JAMA Surgery. 2016;**151**(5):408-415

[21] Svensson JF, Patkova B, Almstrom M, et al. Nonoperative treatment with antibiotics versus surgery for acute nonperforated appendicitis in children. Annals of Surgery. 2015; **261**(1):67-71

[22] Mahida JB, Lodwick DL, Nacion KM, et al. High failure rate of nonoperative management of acute appendicitis with an appendicolith in children. Journal of Pediatric Surgery. 2016;**51**(6):903-911

[23] Pepper VK, Stanfill AB, Pearl RH. Diagnosis and management of pediatric appendicitis, intussusception, and Meckel diverticulum. The Surgical Clinics of North America. 2012; **92**(3):505-526

[24] Goldin AB, Sawin RS, Garrison MM, et al. Aminoglycoside-based triple-antibiotic therapy versus monotherapy for children with ruptured appendicitis. Pediatrics. 2007; **119**:905-911

[25] Lee SL, Islam S, Cassidy LD, et al. Antibiotics and appendicitis in the pediatric population: An American pediatric surgical association outcomes and clinical trials committee systematic review. Journal of Pediatric Surgery. 2010;**45**:2181-2185

[26] McBurney CIV. The incision made in the abdominal wall in cases of appendicitis, with a description of a new method of operating. Annals of Surgery. 1894;**20**:38-43

[27] Jen HC, Shew SB. Laparoscopic versus open appendectomy in children: Outcomes comparison based on a statewide analysis. The Journal of Surgical Research. 2010;**161**(1):13-17

[28] Vegunta RK, Wallace LJ, Switzer DM, et al. Laparoscopic appendectomy in children: Technically feasible and safe in all stages of acute appendicitis. The American Surgeon. 2004;**70**:198-201

[29] Jaschinski T, Mosch C, Eikermann M, et al. Laparoscopic versus open appendectomy in patients with suspected appendicitis: A systematic review of meta-analyses of randomised controlled trials. BMC Gastroenterology. 2015;**15**(1):48

[30] Yau KK, Siu WT, Tang CN, et al. Laparoscopic versus open appendectomy for complicated appendicitis. Journal of the American College of Surgeons. 2007;**205**(1):60-65

[31] St Peter SD, Sharp SW, Holcomb GW III, et al. An evidence-based definition for perforated appendicitis derived from a prospective randomized trial. Journal of Pediatric Surgery. 2008;**43**(12):2242-2245

[32] Hartwich JE, Carter RF, Wolfe L, et al. The effects of irrigation on outcomes in cases of perforated appendicitis in children. The Journal of Surgical Research. 2013;**180**(2):222-225

[33] Simillis C, Symeonides P, Shorthouse AJ, et al. A meta-analysis comparing conservative treatment versus acute appendectomy for complicated appendicitis (abscess or phlegmon). Surgery. 2010;**147**(6):818-829